BREATH OF
THE FOREST

BREATH OF THE FOREST *A Novel*

Copyright © 2025 Lachlan McGregor

First Edition

Printed on paper that remembers being forest

ISBN: 978-91-531-2836-6

Green Scene Publishing

BREATH OF THE FOREST

Lachlan McGregor

A Weary Traveler's Respite

The weight of unread journals pressed harder on Lachlan's shoulders than his overstuffed satchel ever could. He adjusted the leather strap biting into his collarbone, fingers brushing the flask's engraved taniwha monster – its jade eyes worn smooth from a decade of nervous habit. Ahead, the path dissolved into uncertainty, asphalt giving way to moss-capped stones that spiraled upward like vertebrae from the earth. A whiff of cedar cut through the urban haze clinging to his clothes, crisp as a samurai's blade unsheathed after centuries.

His wristwatch beeped – 1:15PM, time to review Henderson's snide commentary on his Yeti microbiota paper. Instead, he stared at a spiderweb spanning two maple saplings, dewdrops arranged along its radial threads like a frozen firework. The leftmost tree leaned at a 72-degree angle, roots breaching the soil in knuckled protest. Zoology whispered in his hindbrain: *Acer palmatum, seasonal defoliation pattern disrupted by—*

A hot resin droplet struck his neck. He swiped at it, fingers coming away amber and fragrant. The scent unspooled a memory: age fourteen, pressed against a cabin window as his father gestured at Tongariro's slopes. "They're not *just* trees, Lachlan. Watch close when the mist rolls in – you'll see the ones that've learned to walk." He'd rolled his eyes then. Now, a cedar's shadow stretched toward him, its feathered branches rustling in a language older than taxonomy.

Three ants trundled across his boot, their bodies translucent under pollen-dusted light. One carried a petal fragment twice its size, purple edges curled like a shōji screen. Against all reason, Lachlan crouched, nose inches from the insect caravan. The petal bearer detoured around a pebble, precise as a Keio line conductor. A laugh bubbled up – not the performative chuckle he used at conferences, but something lighter, younger.

When he stood, the city's murmur had dissolved. Before him, the forest exhaled: leaves susurrating in pentatonic scales, sunlight sieved through canopies to dapple the earth in leaping trout patterns. His satchel hit the ground with a thud, vials clinking protest. First step – cracked magnolia pods released cardamom warmth. Second – fern shadows braille-coded his ankles. Third – a woodpecker's staccato applause from somewhere high above, where branches wove a nave worthy of Chartres.

He didn't notice he'd begun humming until the melody merged with a stream's glissando over stone. Some distant part of his mind, the part that still cared about impact factors and faculty meetings, flickered like a dying bulb. The rest leaned into the wind, tasting the green.

Lachlan's index finger traced the cedar's fissured bark, each ridge a topographical map of droughts survived. "*Cryptomeria japonica*," he murmured, the Latin syllables flattening against wood that had witnessed Shōguns. A ladybug navigated his knuckle's terrain, its shell polished lacquer-red. He held breath – absurdly – as it veered toward a lichen patch the color of oxidized sake cups.

His boots, formerly pounding like judge's gavels, now paused every third step to interrogate wonders: a spider's silk zipline trembling with aphid prey, mica flecks in granite winking conspiratorially, the damp croak of a frog he'd swear wore tiny spectacles. When his cuff snagged on a wild raspberry cane, he found himself apologizing aloud, then grinning at the echo.

The stream found him mid-squat, analyzing fern spore patterns. Light fractured through water into his cupped hands, painting liquid rainbows across life and head lines. Somewhere between sip four and five – oak leaf funnel forgotten on a stone – he noticed his cheeks ached from a decades-unused smile.

"*Hydropsyche angustipennis*," he announced to a moth perched on his knee, then immediately regretted it. The insect's antennae twitched, unimpressed. Lachlan flopped backward, letting leaf detritus reshape his outline. Above, maples braided sunlight through their branches, needles stitching a quilt of gold and emerald. His fingers crept toward a nearby root system, brushing velvety moss that seemed to exhale at the contact.

When did taxonomy become translation? The thought floated up, buoyant as dandelion fluff. A woodpecker answered with morse code laughter.

8

The cedar's bark imprinted a glyph onto Lachlan's forehead. He'd meant to stretch stiff hamstrings, not press himself to the tree like some dendrological groupie. Now the world narrowed to resinous breath and the vascular thrum beneath his palms. A memory detonated: age six, fever-spiked, mother sponging his brow with lavender water. His fingers convulsed against the trunk, expecting recoil. The tree held firm.

Somewhere between breath 12 and eternity, his sternum unlocked with a pop audible to the wren judging from a fern frond. The air turned liquid, photons slowing to syrup-speed as they filtered through needled lattices. When the first tear fell – no, floated – it caught a spider's thread, becoming a prism that fractured light into his closed eyelids.

He emerged marinated in forest hum, legs numb as overproof rum. The flask's weight felt alien now, its contents suddenly garish. Fourteen-year malt met stream with a glugging sigh, droplets pearling on water striders' knees. Across the bank, early fireflies mistook him for kin, their abdomens winking semaphore he almost understood.

Returning, he paused where asphalt reclaimed the land. A streetlamp's sodium glare highlighted trash caught in a storm drain. Lachlan knelt, fishing out a konbini wrapper and a soda can. The acorn in his pocket pressed like a talisman against left ventricle. Ahead, his hotel's neon spat electric vitriol. Behind, the forest held its green tongue. Some choice trembled in the space between.

The Whisper of the Trees

Sunlight pierced the cedar canopy in spears of antique gold, illuminating pollen drifts that swirled like plankton in some arboreal sea. Lachlan's boot crushed a decaying log, releasing spores that danced upward to catch in his beard - six distinct fungal varieties he could name without thinking. The forest's morning breath carried whispers of moss feasting on stone, of spider silk tightening in the mounting humidity, of something deeper his taxonomic vocabulary failed to cage.

His satchel swung like a pendulum against his hip, the brass clasp imprinting its whale motif into his palm as he paused to record three concentric fungi rings on a maple stump. The pen froze mid-sketch. A foreign rhythm threaded through the forest's baseline hum - human respiration syncing with the susurrus of needled branches.

Twenty paces northeast, through a curtain of

hanging moss, a woman stood fused to a cedar's gnarled trunk. Her hiking vest showed REI tags still attached at the cuff, the synthetic fabric jarring against the tree's primordial bark. Lachlan's eyebrows lifted at her posture - forehead bonded to cambium, palms splayed in symmetrical contact, heels dug into loam like grounding rods.

"Excuse me," his voice emerged softer than intended, filtered through layers of green.

The woman's shoulders released incrementally, vertebrae popping like a lock tumbling open. She turned with the deliberate motion of someone reassembling themselves, wisps of salt-and-pepper hair escaping a practical bob. A Stanford alumni ring glinted incongruously on her tree-smeared hand.

"You seek something, yes?" Her English carried the calculated warmth of boardroom negotiations, though the corners of her eyes crinkled with genuine amusement.

"Observing local interaction with biotic communities." Lachlan brandished his notebook like armor. "Dr. Lachlan McGregor, cryptozoology. That is...you're practicing dendrological engagement?"

"Mei Chen. Recovering technocrat." She dusted cedar duff from her Patagonia vest, the corporation's logo half-obscured by a "Certified Forest Therapy Guide" badge. "What your journals call *Shinrin-yoku*, though we're doing proper *Ki no Sasayaki* today."

Lachlan's index finger twitched toward his pen. "Tree Whispering. You mean phytochemical aerosol studies?"

Mei's laugh lines deepened. "Come. This one's been waiting." Her palm met bark with a familiarity that startled him - not a caress, but the firm contact of old friends shoulder-bumping.

Up close, the cedar's scales told stories in fire scars and beetle trails. Lachlan's nostrils flared at the tang of healing resin, his academic cataloging rushing to fill the silence. *Cryptomeria japonica. Estimated age 280 years. Heartwood extract used in traditional anti-inflammator—*

"Forearm tension inhibits reception," Mei noted, adjusting his splayed fingers into a precise arrangement. "Thumbs aligned with radial symmetry, pinkies curled under for grounding. Your left hip needs to..."

A fir cone bounced off Lachlan's shoulder as he contorted into position. The world reduced to cinnamon-hued fissures millimeters from his eyes, the tree's breath warm and resinous against his lips. Somewhere behind him, Mei's voice drifted like wind through reeds.

"Eight generations have pressed here. Samurai wives listening for campaign news. Tea masters seeking water sources. Salarymen..." She paused. "Well. You'll hear."

Lachlan's knee protested the angle. His notebook dug into his ribs, the pen cap leaving a crescent imprint in his palm. Yet as Mei counted breaths in slow Japanese, an unexpected warmth radiated from the bark - not sunlight, but something that pulsed in time with his accelerating heartbeat.

At breath twenty-seven, his calf muscle spasmed. At forty-one, a ladybug navigated the bridge of his nose. By sixty-three, the cedar's vascular rhythm thrummed through his palms, a percussive counterpoint to Mei's steady enumeration.

When the final exhalation misted the trunk, Lachlan staggered back clutching tingling hands. Mei nodded at his trembling fingers.

14

"Tree spoke. You listened."

"But the mechanism..." He rubbed life back into his palms, eyes darting between bark patterns and his useless notebook. "Phloem vibrations? Subdermal piezoelectric response?"

Mei peeled a cedar needle from his collar. "Tomorrow at dawn. Bring better shoes."

As she melted into the green, Lachlan pressed his still-warm palm to the notebook page. The paper absorbed sweat and resin in equal measure, his usually precise script reduced to jagged glyphs: *Tactile phenomena def. external stimuli. Subjective thermal shift...*

The cedar's shadow stretched to engulf his notes. Somewhere overhead, a nuthatch chuckled.

Dawn arrived as a series of gradients - indigo blushing to saffron at the horizon line, frost crystals retreating from sun-warmed stones. Lachlan crouched beneath the cedar with a climber's chalk bag stolen from his luggage, determined to optimize grip conductivity. His field journal lay splayed at the tree's base, pages weighted with river stones and filled with hastily drawn nerve-endings diagrams.

Mei emerged holding two steaming clay cups, her stride still bearing the metronomic precision of boardroom entrances. "Matcha. Caffeine for focus, L-theanine for..." She waved at his chalk-coated fingers. "Whatever this is."

Lachlan wiped green dust on his jeans. "Reducing friction variables. Standardized pressure—"

"Will interfere." She kicked his chalk bag into the underbrush. "Today we work with imperfections."

The ritual began with Mei wiping his palms with bitter-smelling leaves. "*Hinoki* purification. Corporate retreats love this part." Her smile didn't reach the careful part in his hairline as she positioned his thumbs.

At breath thirteen, sweat glued Lachlan's collar to his neck. Mei's counting voice overlapped with his internal monologue:

Hypothesis 1: Delusory tactile feedback from hypoxia Hypothesis 2: Subconscious...

"Eighty-two," Mei corrected, reading his twitching calf muscle.

The cedar's bark shifted beneath his palms - not

texture change, but vibrational frequency. Lachlan's breath hitched as warmth cascaded up his arms like reverse IV drips. His smartwatch buzzed with a stress level notification just as phantom fingers seemed to brush his sternum.

Mei's count pierced the fugue. "One hundred four... five..."

On 108, his hands peeled away with sucking pops. The clearing spun in slow motion - a dragonfly's wings imprinting afterimages, Mei's steaming teacup suspended mid-tilt. Lachlan stared at his palms' spiderweb erythema, the pattern mirroring the cedar's fissures.

"Piloerection," he blurted, rubbing gooseflesh arms. "Adrenergic response to..."

"Tree likes you." Mei pressed her cheek to the trunk. "They prefer listeners to lecturers."

As she disappeared down the trail, Lachlan fumbled for his whiskey flask. The first burn of single-malt failed to eclipse the cedar's lingering presence beneath his skin - not heat, but the glow of a hearth after distant wanderings.

He poured the remaining liquor into moss, watching earth drink where he couldn't. The flask's taniwha stared back, its jade eyes dull against the forest's thrumming verdance.

Rain transformed Lachlan's field notes into a pulpy mass of indecision, the ink bleeding through forty-seven pages of hypotheses to stamp his thighs with temporary dendrological tattoos. He crouched under a makeshift shelter of ferns and regret, watching droplets chase each other down the cedar's ribs to pool where his whiskey flask lay capsized.

Mei materialized holding a lacquered box, her hair escaping its knot in fern-like tendrils. "Your university called. Twice."

Lachlan stabbed at muddy paper. "Tell them I'm dead. Or enlightened. Whichever voids the grant contract."

"Try tea ceremony. Same principle as Whispering." She unrolled tools with surgical precision - bamboo whisk positioned at 32-degree angle, bowl rotated precisely twice before filling.

He snorted. "I don't do placebo."

"Neither does serotonin." Mei's wrist flicked rhythmic circles, foam blooming like alpine peaks. "Twelve-hour workdays. Cortisol showers. When the migraines came..."

Lachlan's pen stilled. Her corporate past materialized between them - power suits hanging in a cedar wardrobe, spreadsheet glow replacing dawn.

The teacup burned his palms familiarly. As steam curled into his nostrils, the cedar's musk intertwined with matcha bitterness. His shoulders dropped half an inch without permission.

At moonrise, Lachlan returned alone to the clearing. His flight ticket tore easily - Osaka to Auckland, tomorrow 10:15AM - the edges catching on bark like ceremonial confetti. Mei's tea bowl made an adequate inkwell for his resignation letter, the characters swirling into abstraction as rain resumed.

When the cedar's first resonance buzzed through his soles at dawn, Lachlan's hands found their mudras without guidance. Somewhere behind closed lids, a taniwha swam through xylem seas, its jade eyes glinting with forgotten potential.

The abandoned flask, now cradling collected rain and cedar needles, sweated condensation onto tenure-track dreams below.

The Call of Nature's Wisdom

Dawn crept through shoji screen ribs, striping the tatami floor with prison-bar shadows that Lachlan's toes avoided instinctively. The cedar's resonance still pulsed through his palms - forty-seven minutes since waking, the phantom warmth defying all circadian logic. He pressed both hands to the floor's reed-woven grid, seeking cool rationality in the precise 90-degree angles. The tatami fought back with splintered whispers of its own origin story - pampas grass sliced, sun-dried, and pressed into domestic submission.

The resignation letter glared up from his travel desk, its corporate watermark visible beneath crossed-out paragraphs. Lachlan's thumbnail dug into the "Dr. McGregor" letterhead, leaving a crescent groove in the paper's throat. Across the room, his open suitcase vomited academic regalia - a Cambridge hoodie's frayed sleeves entangled with hiking boots still caked in sacred Nara mud.

A sparrow collided with the window in an explosion of feather punctuation marks. Lachlan startled, elbow connecting with the whiskey flask that wept condensation onto tenure-track dreams. The taniwha's jade eyes glinted through droplets, its engraved scales warped by curved glass into something amphibiously alive.

He reached for the phone with bark-stained fingers. The rotary dial's clockwise spin mirrored yesterday's cedar mudras as it ate seven digits of institutional purgatory.

"Faculty office. You're aware it's 5AM here?" The department chair's voice arrived coated in antipodean frost.

"I've revised my notice." Lachlan's thumb traced resin circles on the desk. "Requesting sabbatical instead. Two years minimum."

A printer whined in Christchurch. "To chase tree ghosts full-time? Our review board—"

"Phytoncide research intersects with immune response studies. Publishable data on..." He blinked as sunlight hit the abandoned letter, illuminating a coffee ring that spread like mycelium through his signature. "...on interspecies communication methodologies."

The chair's sigh traveled through twelve thousand kilometers of undersea cable. "Your Himalayan Yeti scat analysis was controversial enough."

Outside, wind rearranged maple leaves into temporary kanji. Lachlan's free hand rose unconsciously, fingers splaying in yesterday's bark-press memory. "This isn't cryptozoology. It's...biocultural ethology. The Kyoto Prefectural University's forestry department—"

"Christ, Lachlan. You're fifty-three. Tenure-track positions don't—"

A bead of resin oozed from his palm's lifeline, real or imagined. He brought it to his tongue - sharp as unripe ume, sweet as sap rising. The forest's vascular hum drowned out the chair's droning pragmatism.

"Email the forms," Lachlan interrupted, cedar confidence straightening his spine. "I'll have Shinto shrine keepers co-author. Peer-reviewed animism."

The click echoed like a snapped twig. Through the receiver's cradle, through earthquake-resistant concrete foundations, the mountains called in grandmother pine voices. Lachlan's origami crane - yesterday's abandoned draft transformed - rode thermal currents toward the waiting green.

The hotel room metastasized into a scholar's grove - desk drawers disgorging kanji-inked scrolls that twined with Nature journal PDFs in a helix of competing truths. Lachlan's leather satchel lay eviscerated in the tatami corner, its contents plotting mutiny against organizational conventions. A pressed ginkgo leaf marked page 387 of "Phytoncides and Human Health," its petiole pointing accusingly at the author's outdated sampling methodology.

He attacked the wall with pushpins and washi tape, transforming beige plaster into a living map. Red thread arteries connected ancient cedar groves to his margin notes: "See Hida-Furukawa dendrochronology records 1702 AD - increased resin production during famine years." Blue yarn rivers charted mist migration patterns through the Kii Peninsula's beard-like moss forests. The taniwha flask guarded this fragile ecology from the minibar's plastic ledge, its silver surface fogged with condensation from the ice bucket's last stand.

"Professor Tanaka? Dr. McGregor from..." Lachlan cradled the phone on his shoulder while mopping green tea from a Shinto shrine pamphlet. His big toe absently stroked the map's coastal pine cluster. "Yes, the phytoncide paper was mine. Wondering if your lab does terpene analysis on..."

A cicada screamed through the receiver. "...not a spa researcher," Tanaka snapped. "My work focuses on industrial resin..."

Lachlan trapped the phone under his chin as both hands reconstructed a shrine maiden's tree meditation diagram using sake coasters and cough drop wrappers. "Exactly! Your polymer extraction methods could quantify sacred grove VOC emissions. Imagine calibrating mass specs to detect spiritual experiences!"

Across the room, his hiking boots laughed silently into a moss-stained sock. The whiskey flask sweated in commiseration.

By moonrise, the walls breathed paper. Neon hotel stationery cohabited with 17th-century poetry: "*Misty robes of cedar priests/Draped over mountain's bare shoulders...*" scrawled beside "*See Fig. 3.6 - Cortisol reduction rates.*" Lachlan's fountain pen hovered indecisively over a Venn diagram merging arboreal deities with dendritic cell structures.

The desk telephone rang with Kyoto's dawn. "McGregor," he mumbled around a pencil.

"Shinrin-yoku Association. We received your...unusual proposal." The voice dripped with bureaucratic saké. "Our members don't typically collaborate with foreign..."

He glanced at his big toe, still absently petting the map's paper forest. "I'll take your head priestess sampling terpenes at Nikkō's cedars. Full lab gear under ceremonial robes if needed."

Silence. Then reluctant laughter. "Meet us at Kurama-dera. Come dressed for science and spirits."

The click released him. Lachlan's pen resumed its dance, wedding quantum physics to tree whispering theories in marginalia only a drunk ent could love. Outside, the city's last vending machine glow winked out as his flask yawned empty, ready to be refilled with stranger brews.

The desk lamp's tungsten sun bowed to moonrise, its electric glare retreating from Lachlan's masterpiece. His itinerary unfurled across three tatami mats - a cartographer's fever dream where train schedules dissolved into rhizome networks. Kyoto to Nara bled indigo at the seams, station names overwritten with *"Cryptomeria kami grove (confirmed 4pm) / soil samples required."*

He knelt, cheek pressed to paper, watching lamplight refract through a forgotten cedar resin droplet. The amber lens magnified an inked mountain range into Himalayan proportions, its peaks trembling with each breath. Somewhere beneath "Tuesday: Meet Yuki (tree whispering protocols)", the residue pulsed in time with Nikko's underground hot springs.

"Final approval from Kōyasan's monks," he told the taniwha flask, its engraving now frosted with anticipation. "They want me to sample lichen during morning chant." The silver creature smirked as he uncapped it, pouring a sunbeam's worth of whiskey into hotel glassware.

Lachlan's toast froze mid-arc. Moonlight through the window bisected the liquid, creating dual libations - one for the scientist who'd lectured on phylogenetic bracketing, another for the man who'd recently bowed to an eight-hundred-year-old sugi. The dichotomy burned pleasantly.

His fountain pen hovered over the itinerary's last blank space - a paper clearing between Nagano's birch forests and Yakushima's moss monks. The nib exuded a drop of Berlin-taxonomy black that spread like mycorrhizal networking. From somewhere beyond the window screen, a night heron croaked commentary.

"Alright then," he whispered, pen tip skating across washi. The kanji for "listen" materialized, its radical components dissected into "ear", "king", and the unwritten shadow of "heart".

When the flask finally kissed lips, whiskey carried unexpected notes - petrichor from Nikko's sacred falls, phytoncides from Arashiyama's bent pines, the metallic aftertaste of thirty-seven academic years dissolving. Lachlan's toes curled into tatami, grip tightening on both glass and destiny.

Outside, maple leaves practiced their falling form. Inside, a leather satchel yawned open, hungry for adventures that defied all peer review.

The Forest Guide

The bamboo forest breathed in exhalations of jade light, each stalk a vertical prisoner of its own segmented growth. Lachlan's hiking boots sank into loam that his scientific mind immediately classified - volcanic ash substrate mixed with decaying *Phyllostachys edulis* sheaths. He counted seventeen distinct dew patterns on his left sleeve where mist had condensed, their surface tensions disrupted by wool's hydrophobic fibers. Somewhere beyond the grove's cathedral nave, a temple bell tolled frequencies that made his molars vibrate.

"McGregon-san." The correction came softly as the old man emerged between culms, his wide-brimmed sedge hat catching first light like a parabolic collector. "Not like Scots pine - here, knees bend first."

Lachlan's aborted handshake turned into a bow that nearly toppled his satchel. Three pens and a soil pH meter clattered to the ground as Hiroshi's calloused palms pressed downward, guiding the angle of surrender. Up close, the guide smelled of camphor and fermented tea leaves, his faded windbreaker bearing the ghostly imprint of "Kyoto Forestry Institute, Est. 1983" beneath newer forest therapy badges.

"Your intention," Hiroshi prompted, producing a scroll from his rattan basket. Lachlan stared at the brushed kanji, recognizing only the radical for "wood" repeated like a stuttering pulse.

"To quantify arboreal bioaerosol..." he began, reaching for his spectrometer.

The scroll tapped his wrist with the gentleness of a bamboo whip. "Not here," Hiroshi corrected. "Here." A knotted finger pressed Lachlan's sternum where yesterday's cedar resonance still hummed.

They settled on cross-legged positions that made Lachlan's IT band shriek protest. Hiroshi's breath cycled through four-phase rhythm - 4.7 second inhales followed by 7.3 second exhales, Lachlan's cortex catalogued - while morning light crept up their bodies like a photosynthetic tide. When the first bamboo creak resonated at 132Hz, Lachlan's pen flew open to note: *Compare to Weddell seal trills recorded McMurdo Station '09.*

"Your vessel..." Hiroshi gestured at the trembling pen, "makes waves in still water."

Lachlan pocketed it reluctantly, fingers finding the flask's reptilian contours instead. Three rotations clockwise - his habitual stress response - before realizing Hiroshi's eyes tracked each movement like a botanist noting invasive species.

"Scotch whiskey," Lachlan offered weakly. "For... specimen preservation."

Hiroshi's laugh lines deepened. "My grandfather kept a flask too. For listening to pines during winter." He produced a chipped enamel cup, pouring Lachlan's offering with ceremonial care. The peat smoke aroma mingled unexpectedly with bamboo's chlorophyll punch.

When the bell tolled again, Lachlan startled at the time - 43 minutes had dissolved into light gradients and breath counts. His notebook lay abandoned, its pages fanning gently in the grove's exhalations as Hiroshi pressed a yellowed research paper into his hands. The 1972 Kyoto University text on bamboo allelopathy trembled against his whiskey-damp palms, its margins filled with cursive annotations that blurred scientific jargon into poetry.

Lachlan's boot sole met the grove floor with the subtlety of an excavator, crushing a katydid nymph that launched his conscience into taxonomic guilt - *Tettigonia orientalis, 2nd instar, vital for...* Hiroshi's bare foot flashed alongside, toes splayed to distribute weight across fallen sheaths. Their imprints stared up like mismatched fossil records - Vibram tread versus flesh dendrites.

"Each step," Hiroshi murmured, "is apology to earth." He pressed a hand against bamboo whose ridged surface Lachlan suddenly recognized as vertical braille. The stalk quivered under his palm, transmitting decades of growth spurts and typhoon survivals. His fingers instinctively measured internode spacing - 23.4 centimeters, consistent with optimal...

"Not ruler," Hiroshi chided, adjusting Lachlan's grip into a cradle position. "Grandfather's bamboo."

The flask's slosh timed perfectly with the next breeze-induced creak, liquid pendulum swinging north-northwest as stalks dipped east-southeast. Lachlan's face burned hotter than his abandoned thesis defense. "Apologies, the..."

"Metal tree blood," Hiroshi nodded solemnly before breaking into a grin yellowed like aged parchment. "Mine once carried shochu." He pantomimed youthful staggering between bamboo that Lachlan suddenly saw as sake shop pillars.

Light shifted as clouds breached the grove canopy, photons scattering through Lachlan's eyelashes into prismatic aberrations. Hiroshi's voice floated from somewhere beyond normal auditory range: "Your shadow just married that sapling." Indeed, his elongated silhouette now embraced a young culm, the union trembling as wind rewrote their vows.

When Hiroshi knelt to press cheek against loam, Lachlan followed with creaking joints, his nose meeting a fungal metropolis. Hyphae highways pulsed beneath magnified vision, transporting nutrient caravans between bamboo root terminals. His swab kit emerged reflexively, cotton tip grazing Hiroshi's nostril.

"1997," the old man murmured, inhaling deeply, "smells like the drought year." Lachlan's sterile vial filled with contradictions - decaying cellulose and promise of future growth.

Their parting shadows stretched long fingers across the grove as Lachlan paused to photograph light patterns. Through the viewfinder, Hiroshi's silhouette merged with bamboo until only the sedge hat remained visible - a mushroom cap completing some ancient mycorrhizal pact.

Phytoncides tasted like forgiveness - sharp pinene notes cutting through Lachlan's whiskey palate, limonene softening institutional betrayals. Hiroshi cupped bamboo leaves like a street magician, breathing techniques pulling airborne terpenes into alveolar labyrinths.

"Your machines," he nodded at Lachlan's spectrometer, "count soldiers. We hear general's strategy."

The readout blinked $387\mu g/m^3$ of cis-3-hexenol - crisis communication levels by any botanical standard. Lachlan's pen trembled above the notebook, its ink blending airborne β-phellandrene into permanent record. He suddenly understood medieval monks illuminating manuscripts with beetle shells and oak gall.

"1986," Hiroshi produced a vial of amber liquid, "bamboo's answer to Chernobyl." Lachlan's mass spec would later confirm cesium-137 levels still hovering near background noise.

As afternoon angled through the grove, their tools intermingled - calipers measuring culm diameters while Hiroshi described Meiji-era cultivation songs. The flask passed hand to liver-spotted hand, now containing a tincture of Lagavulin and crushed bamboo shoots that burned like ecological truce.

Lachlan's sabbatical request drafted itself in dappled light, each kanji stroke guided by grove acoustics. When Hiroshi pressed the seal against paper, the bamboo motif stamper left indentations resembling cellular structures.

Departing footsteps carried different weight - left boot sole imprinted with Hiroshi's final gift: a bamboo charcoal insert to filter urban air and academic bitterness. The grove's evening exhalation carried Lachlan's abandoned pen cap, rolling it between stalks until moss claimed custody.

Somewhere above, a black-eared kite screeched equations of lift and drag that no longer required solving. Lachlan's satchel, heavy with scrolls and soil samples, swung in harmonic rhythm with his gait - a pendulum finding its true north between forest and laboratory.

The whiskey flask's new bamboo infusion sloshed gently, its engraved taniwha now wreathed in leafy patterns that almost looked like approval.

Gathering Forest Allies

The teahouse windowsills wore their morning frost like kintsugi cracks, gold-leaf fractures mending night's chill into daylight. Lachlan's pen nib caught on paper fibers, dragging the kanji for "breathe" into a jagged ravine. He scowled at the flawed character, left thumb automatically seeking the cedar resin stain permanently etched into his cuticle - a topographical reminder pressed into flesh during last week's downpour vigil.

His satchel yawned open beside a dregs-crusted teacup, disgorging artifacts across the low table: a spectrometer readout folded into origami crane form, Hiroshi's bamboo charcoal rubbing resembling neuronal pathways, three abandoned invitation drafts annotated with increasingly desperate margin notes ("TONE? TOO CLINICAL - NEEDS MORE... ARBOREAL WHIMSY?"). The current attempt swam before him, ink transforming into tiny root systems that threatened to strangle the phrase "phytoncide exposure benefits."

"Steady on," he muttered, rotating the flask until its taniwha engraving aligned with the tea room's Shinto altar. A dribble of Islay malt christened the final draft - peat smoke mingling with hinoki wood paneling as he recopied the text with surgeon's precision:

The Verdant Accord: A Sylvian Symposium Dr. Lachlan McGregor invites intrepid souls To quantify the ineffable Saturdays at dawn, Yōrō Falls trailhead Metric-based forest bathing & interspecies dialogue Sensibility over skepticism requested

The teahouse owner materialized with fresh matcha, her geta sandals clicking Morse code against floorboards as she examined Lachlan's handiwork. Her sniff conveyed generations of kyō-yasai farmers judging prize radishes. "Foreigners prefer... simpler words." She tapped an announcement for tofu-making workshops.

Lachlan's neck heated. "This isn't ceramic instruction. It's rigorous..." His protest died as she produced a brush pen, transforming his stodgy "symposium" into "joy-wander" with a single fluid stroke.

Outside, the community bulletin board hosted a democracy of desires - lost cats sketched with ukiyo-e flourishes, guitar lessons advertised via chromatic scale mushrooms. Lachlan's thumb found the pine tar plugging a carpenter bee hole as he positioned his notice. The paper curled rebelliously until secured by a lichen-encrusted thumbtack purloined from Hiroshi's grove.

Sudden breeze: Draft #4 detaches Flutters downward like injured swallow Caught mid-air by maple seedling Final draft remains Corner lifting like tree frog's toe pad Adhesive strength insufficient but determined

His boot soles registered the board's vibrations - teenagers approaching, perhaps, or skeptical academics. Instead, a velvet mite ascended the oak frame, its crimson carapace mirroring the stamped wax seal Lachlan had melted from candle ends at 3AM. The creature paused at the meeting coordinates, antennae quivering as if memorizing GPS coordinates.

Lachlan's fingers brushed bark shavings collected in his pocket, their resinous scent triggering sense-memory: Mei adjusting his mudra grip, cedar's heartbeat syncing with carotid pulse. Across the street, seven crows settled power lines into a living staff - their spacing precise as Hiroshi's bamboo measurement intervals.

The taniwha flask warmed against his hip, its silver scales imprinting temporary tattoos through worn denim. Somewhere beyond asphalt and skeptical glances, the forest exhaled through a million stomatal lungs, awaiting calibration.

The forest path recoiled from Sarah's perfume cloud, cedar boughs lifting like offended nobles as she decimated a spider's dewdrop chandelier. Lachlan's field notebook recorded the approach: 94dB footsteps (construction-grade), 23° shoulder tension angle, iPhone generating enough cortisol to sterilize a koi pond.

"You're..." Her gaze swept his mud-caked boots, "...the doctor?" Corporate vernacular armor clanking.

Lachlan's flask hand hesitated mid-offer. "Less clinical trials, more trial-by-arbor."

Sarah's smartwatch illuminated bloodshot capillaries as she silenced alerts. "My EA scheduled this. Frankly, the ROI on..." A nuthatch's territorial trill severed her pitch.

He noted her pupils constricting - not from sunlight filtering through *Cryptomeria*, but the phantom glare of dual monitors. "Your board wants measurable outcomes? Let's calibrate."

Her intake of phytoncides registered as boardroom oxygen - sharp, dangerous. Lachlan's pen tracked her carotid pulse decelerating from 122 to 88 BPM beneath Chantilly lace collar.

"Stress is a non-billable hour," she quipped, but her left thumb worried a Blackberry callus.

The forest retaliated: Hemlock cone impacts shoulder pad Trickles moss slurry down Prada lining Corporate armor breached

Sarah froze mid-email draft (subject line: URGENT - Q3 DEFICITS). Lachlan offered a cedar twig like ceremonial sword. "Your predecessors used these for court petitions. The kami dislike Keynote slides."

Her snort vaporized morning dew. Yet when wind rearranged her chignon into something resembling avian nesting material, Lachlan caught the exact millisecond her mandible unclenched - 11:04:32AM, logged beside sparrow migration patterns.

The taniwha flask passed between them, its

metallic bite overlapped by Sarah's whispered confession: "I haven't missed a quarterly forecast since 2012." The admission pooled at their feet, absorbed by moss trained over centuries in liquid asset management.

The forest attacked Kenji in angstroms, each pollen grain a golden kamikaze breaching nasal citadels. He documented the invasion through watering eyes - humidity 78%, spore density 1423 particles/cm^3, left nostril flow rate approaching whitewater rapids. His grandfather's cracked spectacles (repurposed as magnifiers) transformed a fern's underleaf into Appalachian topography, sori clusters like coal towns clinging to valley ribs.

"Secondary metabolites," came a voice textured like well-oiled calipers. Kenji startled, revealing a coffee stain mapping the Yangtze across his "Immunoboosters 2023" spreadsheet.

Lachlan crouched, smelling of pine pitch and single malt. "Your methodology's sound, but you're missing the volatiles." He brushed the fern, releasing aerosols Kenji's spectrometer pen detected as α-pinene fireworks.

"My granddad knew thirty-seven respiratory

remedies." Kenji's sneeze perfected a jazz scat rhythm. "Died clutching an inhaler anyway."

The flask appeared between them, its taniwha swimming through condensation. "Phytoncides," Lachlan intoned as Kenji sipped, "nature's NK cell orchestra tuning up."

Memories erupted - Grandfather's hands pulverizing mulberry bark, wheezy voice reciting: "Lung wood expands in dampness." Kenji's pen moved unbidden, transforming Lachlan's biochemical discourse into branching diagrams that mirrored both dendritic cells and oak canopies.

A ladybug inspected Kenji's allergen chart, its polka dots echoing the data points. When wind surged through sweet vernal grass, he didn't reach for Kleenex but inhaled the assault - a raw recruit embracing drill sergeant's abuse. Somewhere beyond the snot-damp bandana, his ancestor's ghost nodded approval.

Lachlan's chuckle rumbled like distant wood decay fungi at work. "Next time, ditch the antihistamines. Let the trees prescribe."

Kenji's seventh sneeze of the hour carried a maple samara, its papery wing lodging in Lachlan's beard like a biological post-it. The data point glowed neon in his mind: Allergic rhinitis intensity ⬇ 18% since session commencement.

The sketchpad absorbed Hana's graphite rage, each aggressive stroke snapping charcoal sticks into shrapnel that littered the forest floor like spent artillery. She crouched to retrieve a fragment, fingers smearing yesterday's failed sycamore study across fresh paper - bark texture resolving into the exact shade of Lachlan's whiskey-stained incisor when he smiled.

"Persimmon wood?" His voice arrived filtered through maple leaves, boots avoiding her art supplies with unearned grace.

Hana shielded the sketch - a grotesque caricature of pine needles as prison bars. "Commission work." The lie curdled as Lachlan produced her lost eraser from a pocket, its surface imprinted with incriminating thumbprints and cedar resin.

He studied her abandoned "Urban Canopy" series splayed across moss. "Ah. The 57° perspective trap." His boot toe nudged a sketch of twisted birches. "They prefer oblique angles after monsoon season."

Wind intervened: Page 14 (suffocating willow) lifts skyward Fluttering into hawthorn embrace Exhibited beside actual suffocating willow

Hana's chokehold on professionalism dissolved as Lachlan described Tokyo gallery walls sweating under her climate-controlled landscapes. "They feel... airbrushed," she admitted, charcoal dust confessing what lips couldn't. "Like trees vacuum-sealed for consumer safety."

The flask appeared, its taniwha grinning through condensation. "Try drinking the view." Lachlan's knuckle tapped her latest sketch - a sterile cedar grove. "These trees haven't bled yet."

Hana's sip left peat smoke lingering between molars. When the forest breathed, her next stroke mirrored a branch's arthritic reach, graphite capturing sap's viscous ooze between bark platelets. The paper moaned relief.

Above, a spider lowered itself onto her margin notes, spinning critique silk across the phrase "inauthentic composition." Hana left the annotation intact.

The forest mocked Aisha's Prada mules, their soles rejecting mud's intimacy. She paused beneath a white pine, its branches conducting an orchestra of rustles that resurrected Kampala's jacaranda canopies. A bead of Ugandan sweat (decade-old) escaped her hairline as Lachlan materialized holding a fractured geode - its crystalline teeth mirroring her splintering composure.

"Granite migmatite," he offered. "Earth's nervous breakdown made beautiful."

Aisha's "consultant smile" cracked as her thumb found a scarred cedar trunk. Bark ridges aligned perfectly with childhood memories of tracing banana tree collars. The sob escaped as a botanical term: "Prop roots... they're suffocating in concrete planters back home."

Lachlan's flask paused mid-swig. "Transplant shock," he nodded, dousing the geode until whiskey rivers flooded crystal canyons. "Roots remember what pavements forget."

She pressed palms to pine sap, stickiness erasing months of hand sanitizer. The tree's heartbeat pulsed through her metacarpals - a Lubiri Market drum circle rhythm syncing with carotid flutter. When she finally breathed, phytoncides dissolved Mandarin phrases from her throat, leaving Luganda vowels naked and resonant.

"See? The mugumo fig's bastard cousin." Lachlan tapped a gnarled root, unaware he'd just christened Aisha's first Nairobi apartment view. Her phone buzzed with a developer's demolition notice, screen shattering against pine bark as she embraced arboreal pidgin - half corporate jargon, half agricultural liturgy.

Above them, the last intact silk thread from Aisha's scarf fluttered into a chickadee nest, urban plumage softening hatchlings' worldview.

The forest inhaled in pentameter, drawing five human rhythms into its cadence. Lachlan positioned Hana's sketchpad against a nurse log vibrating at 432Hz - nature's concert A. Kenji's antihistamine bottle rolled into ceremonial position, orange plastic glaring sacrilege against moss velour.

"Intentions," Lachlan prompted, watching Sarah's larynx constrict around unspoken Q3 quotas. The cedar answered first, shedding a scale of bark that landed as ellipsis on her patent leather toe.

Aisha broke first, Luganda verbs tumbling like overripe jackfruit: "Ndagukunda... I used to whisper this to saplings." Her corporate veneer sloughed away, revealing raw nursery rhymes about banana tree lullabies.

Hana's charcoal snapped mid-confession, the fracture echoing through birch stands. "My gallery show... they called it 'sterile deforestation chic'." Paper tears blended with cedar resin, creating accidental pulp art that outshone her thesis work.

Kenji's spreadsheet syntax collapsed into haiku: "Pollen counts lie Grandfather's ghost breathes through bark White blood cells dancing"

Sarah's smartphone chose that moment to vibrate into a fairy ring of destroying angels mushrooms. The S&P update notification died screaming as she ground the device into chlorophyll paste with her stiletto heel.

Lachlan's turn came unbidden, flask raised like sacramental wine. "To the papers we won't publish." The whiskey burned away his last peer-reviewed pretense, leaving only Hiroshi's bamboo mantra humming through his veins.

When the woodpecker's staccato laughter rang out, they mistook it for mockery until realizing - their collective exhalation had shaken loose beetle larvae, providing the bird's first meal. Communion served reciprocal.

The forest issued diplomas in decomposing matter - Sarah's MBA certificate dissolving into a slime mold masterpiece, Kenji's medical charts repurposed as nesting material. Lachlan distributed leaf-patterned cards using Hiroshi's bamboo tweezers, each paper infused with cedar phytoncides that made signatures bloom like startled mushrooms.

Aisha pressed her thumbprint over a laser-printed Uganda, the ink absorbing months of suppressed homesickness until national borders dissolved into root systems. Hana's card developed charcoal sideburns where she'd sketched the group as intertwined saplings, corporate attire sloughing away like bark.

Their procession back to asphalt became an anthropological study - Sarah's blazer abandoned on a hawthorn's outstretched arm, Kenji's sneezes now punctuated with gratitude instead of disgust. At the trailhead vending machine, Aisha inserted yen coins to baptize herself in Pocari Sweat one final time before smashing the "buy" button with her grandmother's pestle technique.

Lachlan remained as twilight reclaimed the cedar, his flask now holding six breath samples and a lock of Hana's charcoal-dusted hair. The taniwha engraving rippled as if swimming through the amalgamated exhalations, his abandoned pager buzzing somewhere in the undergrowth like the forest's newest insect species.

When the first firefly blinked, he answered in Morse: "- .... / .. ... / -. --- - / -- -.-- / .-. . ... . .- .-. -.-. ...." The trees nodded, already drafting their peer review.

Sensory Awakening

The forest edge breathed its own weather system - dawn moisture rising from last night's rain colliding with subway exhaust still clinging to Sarah's blazer seams. Lachlan's boot sole cataloged the transition zone: asphalt melanoma giving way to mycorrhizal networks, his heels crushing urban lichen (*Xanthoria parietina*, thrives on NOx emissions) into sacred humus. His satchel swung pendulum-heavy with Hiroshi's bamboo charcoal inserts and Aisha's confiscated smartphone, its screen still pulsing with phantom board meeting alerts.

"Mind the threshold," Lachlan announced, producing his flask in lieu of a compass. The taniwha engraving wept condensation that mapped altitude sickness across silver scales. Five pairs of eyes followed its arc - Sarah's tracking liquid assets, Kenji's calculating ABV percentages, Hana's noting patina variations worthy of a still life series she'd never exhibit.

A maple key helicoptered into Sarah's french

twist. "We're setting intentions," Lachlan continued, "not Key Performance Indicators." His palm upturned offered three generations of samara wings - 2015's drought-year runts nestled against plump 2023 models. "Let them land where they will."

Kenji's nasal inhaler hissed counterpoint to the forest's first waking breaths. "Like Shinto paper floats?" he asked, adjusting grandfather's spectacles smudged with yesterday's pollen counts. "But measurable?"

"Precisely unmeasurable." Lachlan's thumb released the seeds into a thermal updraft. They rode air currents with stock market unpredictability - one caught in Aisha's silk scarf (Kampala market grade), another skewering Hana's abandoned sketch of the meeting notice board.

Sarah's stiletto excavated a Neolithic midden of bottle caps and acorn shells. "My EA booked this as team-building," she muttered, phone attempting to photograph lichen while recording audio notes. "Nature's supposed to..."

A house centipede traversed her patent leather toe cap. Lachlan watched her breath cycle shift - 6 second inhale (Boardroom Standard) disrupted into jagged 3.4 second gasps. The taniwha flask pressed into her palm delivered 12-year-old peat reek and Hiroshi's bamboo infusion. "Your cortisol's curdling the moss," he whispered.

Twenty-three steps into the forest proper, Hana's charcoal stick surrendered to humidity, weeping across her "Sensory Experience Tracker™". Aisha knelt suddenly, Ugandan soil memory surging through Italian leather soles. "Back home," she murmured, fingers splaying over a termite highway, "we'd say the mugumo fig arrives before the rains."

Lachlan's field notes absorbed her words through the back pocket of hiking pants that still bore stains from Nikko's sacred springs. "Eyes open or closed?" Kenji asked, thermocline meter already probing air strata differences between canopy levels.

The answer came as a velvet mite migration across Sarah's abandoned smartphone, their carmine bodies spelling out "presence" in phylogenetic script only Lachlan's whiskey-soaked cortex could decipher. Somewhere overhead, Hiroshi's borrowed bamboo wind chime tuned itself to A-flat minor - the cedar's preferred resonance.

When the city's last audible ambulance wail

dissolved into nuthatch gossip, Lachlan pressed palms to a lightning-scarred oak. Five human hearts beat counterpoint to xylem pulses as dawn completed its hostile takeover of nightshift shadows.

Sunlight behaved differently here - photons that had survived their 8.3-minute solar journey now diffracting through Sarah's mascara-clumped lashes into prison bar shadows across her tablet. Lachlan noted the exact wavelength ($\approx$560nm) where productivity software blues morphed into maple-shadow greens. "Observe the hopscotch," he whispered, as if coaching novice particle physicists. A Japanese maple leaf descended with calculated whimsy - 2.3 second freefall, rotational speed 47rpm - to eclipse the "Q3 Shortfall" spreadsheet dominating her screen.

The forest chuckled in creek bed cadences. Kenji's cupped hands behind ears formed parabolic dishes harvesting soundscapes - his grandfather's ghost hummed along to the stream's rendition of Sakura variations played on xylophone stones. "Your meter's cheating," Lachlan murmured, displacing the decibel reader with Hiroshi's bamboo listening tube.

Sarah's exhale synchronized with white noise algorithms dying mid-calculation.

At waterside, Aisha's soles rediscovered childhood balance beams - here a granite slab remembering Pleistocene glaciers, there a mossy pipeline remnant from Edo-era sake brewers. Her fingers skimmed liquid that carried molecular whispers of Ugandan downpours, Japanese monsoons, and Lachlan's whiskey flask now cooling in an eddy pool, its taniwha engraving generating microcurrents.

Kenji's Epipen floated forgotten beneath a water strider convention. "The A-flat!" he suddenly crowed, ancestral ear training bypassing corporate tinnitus. A crayfish documented the breakthrough in benthic script. Lachlan's field notes grew damp with revelations – Hana drawing sonar maps of fish bellies, Sarah submerging her wedding ring (Cartier, 2017) to calculate refractive index variations.

The stream performed its alchemy - quarterly reports dissolved into cellulose pulp, a bluegill swallowing PowerPoint bullet points whole. When Sarah's tear followed the watershed cycle (left eye→cheek→jawline→stream→Pacific gyre),

Lachlan's flask intercepted its sodium payload, the alcohol preservative ensuring this particular salinity would outlast civilizations.

Bark doesn't lie. Lachlan's palm met oak cambium in a handshake older than surnames, the tree's frost crack ridges aligning with the scar webbing his knuckles - 1995 chainsaw incident, Waitākere Ranges. "Library access requires proper credentials," he joked weakly, blood memories of white pine sap bandages merging with Kenji's gasp at encountering *Usnea articulata* - Hiroshi's radioactive moss specimen pulsing gently in its dish.

The forest curated its scent archive with pharmaceutical precision. Sarah's Valentino Donna dissolved into component aldehydes, her corporate armor sloughing away to reveal 1998 Biology 101 field trip musk. "It's like..." she breathed, nostrils flaring at loam terroir, "...reverse forensics."

Aisha's braids swung counterpoint to ginkgo root patterns, Kampala's red earth rising through Kyoto's humus to stain her knees sacred. When her pinky grazed a chicken-of-the-woods mushroom, ancestral recipes overwrote takeover bid strategies in neural pathways. Nearby, Hana's charcoal surrendered to humidity, its disintegration rate mirroring abandoned gallery contracts.

In the clearing, seven stones formed a hydrogen bond constellation. Lachlan's flask circulated with ceremonial gravity, whiskey now hosting Kyoto raindrops and Aisha's suppressed homesickness tears. "The cedars..." Kenji began, then sneezed an allergic sonnet that startled a moth into Pollock-esque flight patterns.

As dusk rewrote light parameters, their combined exhalations crafted temporary ice flowers on cedar needles - crystalline art melting faster than stock options vest. Sarah's discarded blazer became mycelium housing, wool fibers accepting spores with more grace than she'd ever shown junior associates. The taniwha flask, now cradling firefly bioluminescence instead of liquor, hummed its approval in F-sharp - the exact pitch of forest twilight in Miyazaki's childhood memories.

The Language of Trees

The path surrendered its arithmetic abruptly
where granite outcrops fractured the forest's
green equations. Lachlan's boot sole registered
the change - volcanic soil pH shifting from 5.4
to 6.1 as they entered the grove's mineral-rich
womb, his collar absorbing the sudden
humidity spike that announced seven ancient
cedars standing sentinel in a geometry
textbooks would reject.

"Circa 1632," he announced, knuckles rapping
a trunk wider than Sarah's corporate limousine
door. "Planted during Tokugawa Iemitsu's
shrine renovations." The cedar wore its scars
proudly - blackened lightning forks preserved
under amber resin cataracts, beetle boreholes
forming braille love letters only woodpeckers
could read.

Hana's charcoal stick hesitated mid-air, its tip
quivering at the grove's asymmetry. "They're..
.leaning." Her artist's eye narrowed at trunks

bent like old samurai backs. "Is that safe?"

"Physics rarely concerns itself with poetry." Lachlan pressed both palms to sun-warmed bark, Yuki's voice resurfacing through cambium layers - *Listen past the xylophone ribs, the real song's in the sapwood's slipstream.* His scars remembered the drill: left palm at 10 o'clock, right at 2, forehead sealant against fissures deep enough to swallow lifetimes.

The demonstration unfolded in biological stereo - Sarah's smartwatch tracking his respiratory rate (12.3 bpm), Kenji's inhaler performing nasal percussion, Aisha's silk scarf snagging on a Kapok pod's cottony rebellion. At breath seventeen, the cedar's vascular thrum bypassed Lachlan's medulla, syncing directly with the whiskey tremor in his hands.

"Your turn." He peeled away reluctantly, bark ridges leaving temporary dendroglyphs on his skin.

Sarah approached her chosen tree like hostile merger. "Optimal contact surface area?" Her blazer's shoulder pads compressed moss into memory foam as she calculated angles.

"Instinct over spreadsheets," Lachlan advised,

watching Hana's charcoal assault paper with jagged strokes that captured the cedar's disdain.

Aisha's cross-legged posture dissolved three times - left knee bouncing to imaginary Outlook alerts, fingers drumming supply chain optimizations into fern beds. When kapok fibers drifted across her nostrils, she startled at phantom memory of Kampala's drought-season winds carrying identical parachute seeds.

Kenji alone achieved symmetry - grandfather's spectacles fogging with each measured exhale, allergic rhinitis temporarily muted by the cedar's antimicrobial sigh. His notebook lay abandoned, pen rolling downhill to baptize itself in a rivulet of last night's rain.

"Bullshit." Hana's charcoal snapped against gnarled roots, powdered carbon blooming across sap flows older than her great-grandmother's art school diploma. "It's just cellulose and photosynthesis."

Lachlan pocketed the broken charcoal, fingers emerging stained with rebellion. "Van Gogh called stars his nervous system. What's your cedar's diagnosis?"

Above them, a nuthatch performed quality control on Sarah's breathing technique, dropping an acorn cap that landed precisely where her spreadsheet predicted heart rate variability should peak. The forest held its multiple-choice exam - one part phytoncide elixir, two parts humbled human sweat.

Lachlan's flask caught the panic in prismatic refraction - Hana's fifth abandoned sketch fluttering groundward, its cubist cedar dissolving into charcoal rage at the precise angle needed to blind Sarah's solar-powered calculator. The grove breathed its patients' chart: elevated cortisol in the western quadrant, restless legs syndrome due southeast, one anomalous steady pulse beneath the grandfather pine.

He intercepted Hana mid-stomp, her boot hovering over a slime mold busily converting anger vibrations into fruiting bodies. "Your lines," he murmured, catching a charcoal shard mid-fall, "they echo the tree's teenage growth spurt."

"Bull." Her glare ricocheted off dendrochronology maps in his open journal. "You can't anthropomorphize cellulose."

"Can't I?" Lachlan pressed her palm to a burl

shaped like Einstein's cerebellum. "This one survived the 1707 Hoei eruption by growing asymmetrically. Sound familiar?"

Aisha's meditation unraveled thirty feet east, Ugandan Swahili blending with supply chain jargon as her fingers compulsively swiped at non-existent phone alerts. "Mkutano wa Jumatatu...quarterly projections...nahitaji kupiga simu..." A falling sweetgum leaf arranged itself into bullet points across her lap.

Sarah's tablet beeped calamity - mold spores colonizing the charging port as she input variables for "arboreal connection intensity." "If we quantify phytoncide uptake," she lectured a disinterested woodlouse, "we could benchmark against Nordic forest bathing studies."

Only Kenji flowed river-smooth, grandfather's pocket watch (1907 Seikosha, radium dial) ticking counterpoint to cedar's resinous pulse. The antihistamine tablet dissolved beneath his tongue released generations of folk wisdom - mugwort tea steeped in hand-forged iron kettles, persimmon leaf poultices applied by hands still smelling of Meiji-era printer's ink.

"Try sketching the roots you can't see," Lachlan suggested, pressing Hana's charcoal against paper mottled with slime mold's yellow tendrils. "The mycelium marketplace down there makes Wall Street look civilized."

Aisha startled at phantom buzzes, her empty pocket producing phantom board meeting terrors. When a cicada's drone synchronized with Kampala's rainy season downpour memory, she accidentally snapped a twig still humming with last night's aphid rave.

Sarah's spreadsheet glitched magnificently - cells merging into chlorophyll green as lichen claimed her tablet's edges. "This methodology.. ." she protested weakly, fingers brushing decay patterns that mirrored Q3's failed marketing metrics.

Lachlan's confession emerged unbidden, watered by cedar shadow and Hana's glare. "Yuki laughed when I arrived with spectrometer arrays. Said my machines couldn't hear the trees' bass register." His thumb rubbed the flask's taniwha, scales worn smooth by a decade of similar admissions.

Kenji's cedar chose that moment to release a pollen plume directly into his sinuses. Instead of sneezing, he inhaled generations of peasant wisdom - grandfather's voice layered over forest hum: *Allergy is just intimacy pursued too fast.*

The forest dialed up its amplifier as Lachlan distributed pine-resin earplugs - Tokyo's skyline dissolved into tympanic membrane, Sarah's stiletto lost its staccato punctuation, and somewhere beyond the seventh cedar's buttress roots, the first tremors of communion began brewing in Kenji's metacarpals like long-fermented sake finally achieving perfect rice-to-koji balance.

"Choose one sense and break its leash," Lachlan instructed, pressing Sarah's palm against resin ooze that smelled suspiciously like her kindergarten's finger-paint cabinet. Aisha's scarab bracelet hummed against Ugandan pulse points, its bronze wings remembering desert crossings older than corporate mergers.

Kenji's cedars decided to speak in grandfather's dialect - a subcutaneous rumble traveling from toenails to occipital ridge that bypassed Western medicine's entire pharmacopeia. When the third vibration wave hit, his Seikosha watch spun madly before settling into perfect sync with the tree's sugar transport rhythm.

"I-it's...translating!" His fingers fluttered bat-like against bark, charting sap flow through epidermal braille. "Like a server room's coolant system, but organic!"

The grove approved in fractal patterns - Sarah's abandoned tablet sprouting lichen bar graphs, Hana's charcoal liquefying into xylem-inspired gradients. Aisha's bullet-point leaf rearranged itself into Swahili proverbs about baobab wisdom.

"Again, slower," Lachlan urged, hiding his trembling hands behind Hiroshi's bamboo flask. Kenji's cedar obliged with a subsonic purr that unknotted Aisha's shoulder muscles and temporarily erased Hana's art school debt stress.

Sarah's nose led the rebellion next - phytoncides hijacking her olfactory bulb to replay the exact Crayola carnation pink scent from her first uncontaminated creativity. Her spreadsheet addiction dissolved somewhere between pine ester emissions and the sudden craving for sidewalk chalk.

Hana's surrender came coated in graphite. "Fine. But if this ruins the composition..." Her forehead met bark with force enough to startle a nut-weevil symphony into dissonance. The forest answered through paper grain - sketchpad fibers aligning into rootlet patterns that bypassed her cynical cortex entirely.

By the time the cicadas shifted key signatures, even Sarah's smartwatch had converted to forest time - its minute-hand jitter replaced by the stately progression of shadows climbing cedar flanks. Lachlan's abandoned pager, still buzzing somewhere under blackberry brambles, finally ran out of battery mid-alert.

The taniwha flask lay empty but content, its silver scales tarnished with fingerprints from every failed and triumphant attempt. As afternoon light performed its final gilding of the grove's cathedral arches, Kenji's cedar deposited a single scale insect on his collar - nature's version of a participation trophy, still humming with the afterglow of connection.

The Joy of Forest Craft

The cedars surrendered their hold reluctantly, birthing the group into a grove where sunlight fell like discarded puzzle pieces. Lachlan's boot sole registered the precise moment volcanic grit yielded to alluvial silk - 6.2pH to 5.8, a gradient even Sarah's starched blazer couldn't defy. He watched maple keys helicopter into her French twist, their flight paths mocking the abandoned tablet's predictive algorithms. Somewhere west, the taniwha flask's remaining whiskey wept condensation into moss that remembered Shōgun processions.

"Mindful crafting," Lachlan announced, pressing an oak gall to his ear like seashell resonance, "requires forgetting what museums taught you." His thumb traced the gall's tumorous contours - nature's pottery wheel spun by chemical betrayal. Sarah's pen hovered over a pocket Moleskine, its pages already cross-referenced with Nordic forest bathing studies. She cataloged leaf venation patterns with the intensity of an FDA auditor.

Kenji crouched like samurai examining battlefield terrain, grandfather's watch chain dragging through loam.

His inhaler hissed counterpoint to the stone selection ritual: 7.3 seconds per pebble, quartz density measured against Meiji-era asthma diaries. "This one," he murmured, polishing an andesite fragment, "contains Mount Hiei's 1708 eruption chronology."

A gust rearranged Hana's charcoal bangs as her fingers hovered above a birch scroll curled tighter than gallery contracts. The bark's parchment texture triggered muscle memory - Art Center critiques, professors dissecting her margins. A woodpecker's morse code suddenly synced with her radial pulse, stabilizing the tremor in her collecting hand. She snapped the bark free with a crack that sent seven tree runners scrambling.

"Marvelous!" Lachlan materialized behind her, flask imprinting temporary scales on the birch. "That's the spirit Hiroshi's bamboo grove tried teaching me." His palm upturned revealed three acorn caps brimming with last night's rain - natural sake cups clinking promises.

Aisha's scarab bracelet caught midmorning light as she rotated a pine cone, its spiral pattern mirroring her Kampala estate's driveway. The resin scent unspooled memories: eight years old, smuggling fig sap past security to make dollhouse furniture. Her pinky tested the cone's gummy tears, viscosity matching 1998's drought-year harvest. When the third scale released unexpectedly, she laughed - a sound foreign as the green lacewing landing on her collar.

Sarah's tablet beeped calamity from its fern reliquary. "If we standardize collection parameters..." Her blazer sleeve snagged on hawthorn, transforming into a reluctant basket for crimson berries. "Weight ratios between organic matter types could optimize..."

"Ah, but the forest hates optimization." Lachlan pirouetted through sunbeams, demonstrating how sword ferns make better calligraphy brushes than Pilot pens. A Japanese marten paused mid-hunt to judge his technique. "That mandala you're drafting in your head? It's already growing underfoot." He stamped, releasing a cloud of springtail performers from the soil stage.

Kenji's sixteenth stone clicked into place, an

igneous timeline spanning Fuji's birth to Hiroshi's childhood. His sneeze scattered the chronology, creating accidental artistry that mirrored grandfather's final charcoal sketch. "Unsanitary," he sniffed, though his eyes lingered on the pattern's perfect asymmetry.

Aisha's pine cone escaped custody, rolling downhill to become an ant army's siege engine. She gave chase, silk scarf capturing seven grasshopper hitchhikers. When the cone lodged between cedar roots, she shrugged and began constructing a bark ramp, tongue poking through teeth like third-grade trigonometry days. The ants waved antennae in what might've been thanks.

Hana's birch scroll unfurled ghostly white against mossy parchment. Charcoal trembled, then dove, chasing beetle trails that mocked straight lines. Somewhere between a bark beetle's love letter and the woodpecker's critique, her shoulders forgot their gallery hunch. The resulting spiral might have offended her professors - and for the first time, she hoped it did.

Sarah's berry-stained blazer sagged under pine cone ballistics and Kenji's volcanic timeline. Her tablet screen faded into lichen mosaic, battery icon flashing like a samurai's dying breath. When a crane fly landed on the "OPTIMIZE" prompt, she didn't swat it, but watched legs trace dendrite patterns across dead pixels.

Lachlan's flask found temporary rest atop a nurse log, its taniwha engraving eyeing the proceedings. Below, slime mold explored the stainless steel curves, tasting centuries of Islay peat and Hiroshi's bamboo grove desperation. The forest leaned closer, breathing phytoncide fog over collected treasures - maple wings, stone chronicles, birch scrolls, and one hijacked blazer becoming something textbooks wouldn't recognize.

The clearing inhaled as knees met earth, seven sacred geometry apprentices unaware they worshipped at the altar of chaos theory. Lachlan's flask sweated circles on a nurse log where slime mold plotted its next infiltration vector. Sarah's "organized" materials formed a color-coded siege against entropy, while Aisha's pine cone lay mid-roll like a dice deciding their fates. Somewhere beneath them, the forest's mycelium network placed bets in hyphae sign language.

Hana's birch scroll crackled open, revealing beetle script annotations. Her charcoal hovered - art school critiques echoing ("Too derivative of Mondrian's necrophilia!") - until a nuthatch's upside-down scrutiny shamed her into the first stroke. The stick landed askew, its asymmetry triggering allergic reactions in her muscle memory. She reached to correct it, but Lachlan's whiskey breath whispered: "Let it colonize the space first."

Sarah's protractor bisected the forest floor into tax brackets. Maple leaves sorted by spectral reflectance values formed a corporate rainbow missing only the PowerPoint arrow. "Symmetry reduces variables," she informed a confused earthworm, unaware her berry-stained blazer now mirrored the fall foliage color wheel.

Kenji's stones clicked like grandfather's abacus beads. Andesite bronchi branched into pumice alveoli, his inhaler canister forming a diaphragm that pumped imaginary phytoncides. When a beetle disrupted the hierarchy, he gasped - then leaned in, documenting how chitinous legs completed the circulatory metaphor.

Aisha's pine cone made its break during an argument between two chickadees. Rolling past

Sarah's leaf ghetto, it caromed off Lachlan's flask into Kenji's pulmonary masterpiece. She froze, corporate apology rising, but the stones' new configuration suggested something wiser than lungs. Her giggles startled a moth into pollinating Hana's self-doubt.

"Magnificent impermanence!" Lachlan crowed, stealing a stone from Kenji's masterpiece to scratch moss into Hana's margins. His thumbprint analysis of a wilting leaf became accidental body art - chlorophyll tattoos mapping vascular regrets.

By noon, the mandalas bled into each other like drunken watercolors. Sarah's spreadsheet, abandoned to slug renovations, transformed into bark pulp under Aisha's scarab bracelet pendulum. Kenji's grandfather's watch found new purpose timing lichen growth across his inhaler chain. Hana's sticks, once prisoners of perpendicular angst, now radiated in supernova formation fueled by stolen moss and beetle approval.

Lachlan's flask, emptied of everything except three ladybug stowaways, conducted the chaos like a whiskey-soaked metronome. The taniwha smirked as the forest redrew their human borders - termite engineers adjusting angles, spider silk connecting disparate elements, and one pine cone completing its revolution into collective genius.

The mandalas grew borders in twilight, their edges blurring like drunk monks' calligraphy. Lachlan's flask lay exhausted, its taniwha now moss-bearded from slime mold attentions. Hana's spiral pulsed like exposed tree rings, each revolution counting gallery rejections and beetle approbations in equal measure. Somewhere beyond the clearing, the forest held its breath, waiting to see if humans could finally speak its love language.

Sarah knelt first, berry-stained fingers tracing where her leaf taxonomy had been reinvented by invertebrates. "They improved the hierarchy," she admitted, watching an earwig rearrange color gradients with military precision. Her protractor floated in a fern-choked puddle, compass point rusting into oblivion.

Aisha's scarf cradled Kampala in lichen and pine cone outriggers. "My father called forests inefficient," she whispered, as a spider spun silk bridges between acorn capitals. "But look.. ." Her pinky touched a dewdrop mirror reflecting both scarab bracelet and stranger's smile.

Kenji's stone lungs billowed with ant cargo, inhaler canister now hosting a violet sprout. "Grandfather's watch," he realized, "finally matches the trees' clock." The timepiece showed 1947, the year his ancestor first prescribed moss poultices for factory lung.

Hana's charcoal spiral had birthed mushroom constellations. "They told me abstraction required distance," she laughed, smearing soot to correct a beetle's overreach. The woodpecker returned, chiseling approval ratings into adjacent birch.

Lachlan poured his last drops into the communal canvas. "Mei's first looked like a drunken hedgehog," he confessed as whiskey merged with slug trails. "But the cedars recognized the effort." His palms pressed earth, transferring bark glyphs learned through three failed sabbaticals.

At moonrise, the mandalas became one. Sarah's berry fingerprints merged with Kenji's volcanic timeline, Hana's soot spiral cradling Aisha's scarab archipelago. The forest exhaled its verdict through owl feather brushes and moth-wing erasers, perfecting edges only darkness could comprehend.

When the taniwha flask finally rolled empty, it carried new engravings - lichen signatures, ant routes, and the faintest ghost of corporate perfume. Somewhere beyond sightlines, seven cedar saplings leaned closer, memorizing human patterns for future whispering.

Weathering the Storm

The forest held its breath in that peculiar stillness Lachlan's joints recognized before memory did - left pinky twinging where a Rotorua landslide had cracked it in '03, phantom weathervane. Above, cumulonimbus armadas massed beyond the canopy's green demilitarized zone, their undersides bruising from pearl-gray to the purple-black of oversteeped hōjicha. Sarah's tablet chirped behind him, its doppler radar animations flattening atmospheric rebellion into candy-colored blobs.

"Dr. McGregor?" Her Louboutin heels sank into pathside muck, each syllable clipped for boardroom consumption. "The NTT weather satellite shows precipitation probabilities at—"

"Ninety-seven and three tenths percent," Lachlan finished, nostrils flaring at the ozone tang rolling downslope. Somewhere beyond the treeline, a juvenile cedar released terpene screams only storm-sensitized resin ducts could parse. He turned, noting Mei's white-knuckled grip on her Forest Therapy First Aid kit and Kenji's experimental rain gauge already collecting anticipatory dew.

Sarah's French cuff snagged on blackberry bramble, Burberry trench gathering fern spores like a billionaire's version of beggar's lice. "We should postpone. The liability waivers don't cover—"

Lachlan's laugh startled a nuthatch into Morse-code alarm calls. "Ever seen lightning dance across Nikko's gold-leaf shrines? The gods put on their best shows when insurance lapses." His thumb found the taniwha flask, its engraved scales prickling with static.

First raindrop impacted Sarah's tablet at 10:47:23 JST, the splash refracting corporate spreadsheets into fractal irrelevance. She recoiled as if acid-spattered, silk blouse absorbing the assault's molecular history - Cretaceous seawater, Hanford nuclear runoff, Shinto shrine purification sprinkles.

Kenji's grandfather's barometer confirmed reality with mercury-smooth certainty. "Pressure's dropping like the '23 Kanto quake readings." His Nikon began rapid-fire documentation of leaves flipping silver under pregnant droplets.

Mei's certification manuals rustled in protest from her guide-pack. "Standard protocols require shelter when—"

"Protocols?" Lachlan spread arms wide as a shiitake-log deity, rain speckling his salt-and-whiskey beard. "Your corporate retreats never taught how cryptomeria resins liquify during storms? The real terpene fireworks?"

Aisha sneezed monsoon memories - Kampala's red clay rivulets carrying childhood toys to Lake Victoria. Her Prada mules, caked in sacred Nara mud, suddenly made profound sense. "In Uganda, we'd say the sky is shedding its bark."

Hana's sketchbook pages puckered like offended bureaucrats. She hunched protectively over a half-finished cedar study, charcoal lines dissolving into Rorschach storms. "My commission requires dry media specs!"

Lachlan scooped a marble-sized hailstone mid-fall. "Tell your clients truth has a humidity clause." He popped the ice between molars, crunching centuries-old atmospheric particulates. "Coming?"

The forest answered first - woodpecker drumrolls from lightning-rod pines, spiderlings ballooning into the gale like eight-eyed paratroopers. Sarah clutched dead tablet to chest, its Apple logo dribbling electrolytic tears onto Gucci zebra-print sleeves. Mei's emergency whistle bounced against sternum in time with quickening heartbeat.

They advanced as the canopy's drum section unleashed its opening number, Lachlan's boots syncopating puddles into Jacobean galliards while Kenji's light meter documented the precise lux value of dread becoming wonder. Somewhere beyond the downpour's white noise, a forgotten girl in a Silicon Valley cubicle lifted her face toward emergency sprinklers and laughed.

Shelter arrived as a dendritic cathedral - an eight-century-old oak whose bark wealed with Edo-period sword tests and firework scars from MacArthur's victory parades. Lachlan pressed his whiskey flask to a deep cleave in its trunk as if taking communion. "Met a daimyo's ghost here in '98," he shouted over the deluge. "His armor still smelled of wet lacquer and regret!"

Sarah folded her wrecked jacket into a sodden Rorschach cushion, the garment's DNA now 3% Nara topsoil. "This is exactly why we have indoor team-building exercises." A shiver betrayed her, trailing goosebumps down corporate-approved posture.

Mei's pulse oximeter clipped onto Kenji's finger with clinical precision. "97% saturation. Elevated but within—" Her certification charts drowned mid-sentence as thunder detonated directly overhead, shaking free a shower of acorn caps and samurai-era nails from the oak's upper chambers.

Aisha's palms flew to ears, her mother's monsoon lullaby ("Mvua kubwa, roho kubwa") surfacing through muscle memory. Kenji's hydrophone captured the exact moment her hum synced with a raindrop's impact on wisteria leaf below - 132Hz, the frequency of Ugandan thumb pianos tuned for rain dances.

"Sensory deprivation's overrated!" Lachlan bellowed, stripping socks to wring them over the oak's thirsty surface roots. "Let your cortex process the chaos!" His big toe pointed to where Hana's disintegrating sketchbook bled Rembrandt-dark streams into moss. "There's your commission's soul, laid bare!"

Mei's disaster protocols drowned in the storm's arrhythmia. She pressed both palms to the oak's northeast face, fingers finding grooves where seven generations of shrine carpenters tested their chisels. The bark breathed its biography - saké spilled during Taishō-era festivals, shrapnel shards from B-29 strafing runs, the slow cancer of 1970s acid rain.

Sarah's Rolex fogged under the humidity, its Swiss gears no match for a samara seed's helicopter descent onto her bare forearm. "These are sterile environments!" she protested weakly as Lachlan guided her palm to the oak's gnarled burl.

"Tell that to the penicillin factory in your shoes." His thumb traced concentric circles on the burl's tumorous surface. "This fellow started life as a samurai's arrow injury. Made peace with the insult centuries back."

Kenji's parabolic mic isolated a raindrop's journey - maple leaf (high C), fern frond (F-sharp), cedar twig (vibrato guttural hum). His spectrogram app crashed under the data load, leaving only the oak's interpretation: a lullaby in Lydian mode that Aisha harmonized through chattering teeth.

Hana's charcoal surrendered its carbon soul to rainwater, swirls resolving into something bold and preliterate. She sketched the oak's scars with a broken umbrella rib, each stroke validated by thunder's timpani.

When lightning backlit the forest in magnesium-white revelation, Sarah's pupils contracted to boardroom-presentation dot points. Then widened. "I used to..." A laugh bubbled up, unbossed and unmanaged. "There was this parking lot sprinkler in Brentwood..." Her stockinged feet hit the downpour, each toe reveling in mud's vulgar squelch. Mei's emergency blanket rustled uselessly as the storm sang its aria of impermanence.

Above them, the oak's crown jewels - last season's abandoned oriole nest, a Shinto prayer board fragment, Lachlan's favorite whiskey cap - danced their rain-soaked jig. Somewhere beyond the tempest, the ghost of a corporate wellness consultant wept at the sight.

Light fractured into alchemical wonder as the downpour relented, water's lens revealing the forest's clandestine chromatic congress. Kenji's camera shuddered against his nose bridge, autofocus overwhelmed by a dewdrop magnifying moss reproductive structures into jade-green launchpads. "The sporophytes! They're...they're helical!" His whisper stirred air molecules still trembling from thunder's basso profundo.

Lachlan pressed Sarah's palm against cedar bark sodden as a sailor's grave marker. "Feel those ridges? Each a drought year's journal entry." Her French-tipped nail traced growth rings swollen with monsoon memory, cuticle collecting lignan secrets older than her divorce proceedings.

Aisha's toes breached loam's surface tension, Kampala's red earth rising through Kyoto's volcanic ash substrate to stain her soles ancestral crimson. "We'd make rain harps from banana fibers," she murmured, kneading mud between metatarsals with motions remembered from grandmother's pottery wheel.

Mei's air quality monitor beeped contrapuntal to dripping branches. "PM2.5 levels dropped 62% since..." Her voice trailed off as a spider's storm-repaired web glinted with prismatic contempt for quantification.

"Over here!" Sarah's corporate bark softened to playground wonder. A fallen log hosted a coven of *Mycena luxaeterna*, their bioluminescent gills pulsing urgent semaphore. She crouched, blouse sleeve absorbing luminous ooze. "They look like...like..."

"Your seventh birthday sparklers," Lachlan finished, conjuring Santa Monica beach evenings where divorced parents' arguments dissolved in pyrotechnic sulfur. Sarah's nod sent a childhood tear mixing with mushroom dew.

Hana's charcoal met rainwater in unholy matrimony, the slurry cascading across her sketchbook's surviving pages to birth Rorschachian giants. "They told us at RISD," she muttered, wrist rotating like an exorcised clockwork, "controlled washes require sable brushes and—"

"Bollocks," Lachlan declared, flinging a pine cone through her masterpiece. "Van Gogh used house paints and desperation." The projectile's wake birthed accidental negative space that made the mushrooms sing.

Kenji's spectrometer app pinged. "The indigo shadow spectrum matches Fukushima's morning glory mutations!" His excitement scattered a snail's meticulous trail, the mollusk responding with accelerated mucus production.

The gratitude circle formed where lightning had forged instantaneous wetlands. Mei clutched her certification badge like rosary beads until a dragonfly's landing transferred sacred iridescence to its plastic veneer.

"Forgot how mud squelches between toes," Aisha began. Sarah's "Bioluminescent time capsules" overlapped Kenji's "Hyphae fiber optics." Hana's charcoal-stained fingers signed liquid grace notes in the humid air.

When the rainbow's arrival silenced them, its arc cradling the forest in fugitive refraction, even Lachlan's whisky-cured tongue found no words. The taniwha flask, refilled with jewel-bright runoff, approved their vow of silence.

The forest released them changed - Sarah's blouse sleeve blooming lichen medals, Kenji's glasses framing eyes widened three aperture stops, Aisha's braids threaded with oak gall ink tendrils. Lachlan's boots left leaden prints in the retreating mud, his whiskey compass pointing toward Arashiyama's contested watersheds.

"Hold this," Hana commanded, thrusting her disintegrating sketchbook at Mei. Pages floated earthward like arboreal ash, each rain-warped stroke colonized by beetle calligraphy and Kenji's spectrometer data. The forest service manual in Mei's pack absorbed charcoal shadows, transforming into a hybrid scripture.

"Hokusai meets data viz," Sarah observed, her Rolex fogging permanently at 11:47 - the hour her divorce papers had been signed. She added a thumbprint smudge that completed a mycelium network's missing node.

Kenji's triumphant shout bounced off cedar stands. Beneath the sheltering oak's root knob, spring rains had exhumed a moss-crusted plaque: *For Lord Kuroda's Loyal Steed - Fell During the Great Tempest of 1682*. The engraved characters swam with centuries of xylem and Lachlan's single-malt libation.

Aisha's fingers recalled ancestral weaving patterns as she bound resurrection fern into her hair. "In Kampala," she said, plaiting faster than corporate meeting minutes, "we wore storms as crowns."

Their exit procession became a palimpsest of ingress - Sarah's barefoot prints overwriting stiletto divots, Kenji's equipment bag shedding lenses into trailside ferns, Mei's emergency blanket repurposed as fungal spore collector.

At the parking lot's edge, cicadas rasped a mocking farewell. Sarah's waterlogged iPhone shuddered to life in her mud-caked purse, its screen cracked into a mandala that improved the stock ticker display. She left it buzzing beneath a stone carved with weather-worn kanji even Lachlan couldn't parse.

"The Nikkei will survive without you," he assured, pressing a cedar-sap-stained itinerary into her palm - *Shirakami-Sanchi: UNESCO Site. Oldest Beech Forest in Asia. No Cell Reception.*

As Hana's collaborative sketchbook disintegrated into a mycorrhizal masterpiece behind them, the taniwha flask's new contents sloshed approvingly. Somewhere beyond the tree line, seven cedars adjusted their growth trajectories by 0.3 degrees - the exact angle of human hearts cracking open.

Personal Forest Histories

The forest steamed its surrender to the departed storm, every frond and fern performing evaporative alchemy that misted Lachlan's eyelashes with liquid prismatics. His boots squelched through mud still protesting its quick-draining volcanic substrate, the air thick with ionized oxygen that made Sarah's corporate perfume curdle into something chemical and sad. Ahead, the clearing exhaled through veils of rising vapor - seven moss-draped stones emerging like the vertebrae of some primordial beast drowned in chlorophyll.

Lachlan's thumb found the bamboo measuring rod Hiroshi had pressed into his palm last equinox, its surface notched with 108 grooves for sacred alignments. "Mind the *Selaginella*," he cautioned, watching Aisha's mules threaten a patch of spike moss that had survived since Edo-period landscaping. His rod tapped stone #3 - warm andesite veined with plagioclase streaks - adjusting its position three centimeters westward to honor the Kii Peninsula's geomantic traditions.

The talking stone emerged from his satchel's whiskey-scented depths, its ovoid form worn smooth by Miocene tides and countless anxious palms. Cretaceous fossils swirled beneath the surface - ammonite whorls fossilized mid-flight, belemnite guards pointing accusations at modern intruders. Sarah accepted it first, her thumbnail digging into a coccolithophore graveyard as the group settled into silence thick as udon dough.

Above, a varied tit paused mid-forage, wings half-spread in avian semaphore. Lachlan counted the interval - 5.2 seconds of stillness mirroring Sarah's respiratory hesitation - before her knuckle cracked against Jurassic limestone inclusions.

"Family camping trip," she began, voice calibrated for shareholder meetings. "Adirondacks, 1998." A bull-headed ant traversed her ankle, retracing the path of long-dead scouts who'd explored her eight-year-old sneakers. Lachlan noted how her clavicle shadows deepened with each confession - 23% opacity increase correlating with pineal gland activation.

Kenji's nose twitched at the word "nightmares", his grandfather's herb pouch producing a stealthy whiff of mitsuba leaves. Across the circle, Hana's charcoal-smudged nail traced bryophyte patterns that mirrored her abandoned Tokyo skyline sketches. The forest leaned closer - wood fern fronds tilting parabolic ears, a redback spider suspending silk production to monitor human vulnerability.

Lachlan's flask warmed against his thigh, its taniwha engraving pressing scales into denim like ritual scarification. He remembered the Kyoto circle where salarymen's confessions had evaporated faster than morning dew, their trauma sealed beneath laminated business cards. But here, Sarah's stone passed hand to trembling hand, each transfer depositing microdermal truths into the clearing's mycorrhizal network.

As Kenji's turn approached, a shrike's hunting cry severed the stillness - three staccato notes echoing the herb pouch's drawstring being tugged. Somewhere beneath them, the moss drank deeply, its capillary action siphoning shame and jasmine tea residue with equal biological indifference.

The talking stone chilled in Sarah's palms like glacial till, its Precambrian feldspar veins conducting remembered frost from that Adirondack October. Her thumb circled a zircon inclusion - 1.2 billion-year-old time capsule outlasting both dinosaurs and divorce settlements. Somewhere beneath the moss, mycelium trembled at the cortisol sweat beading her hairline.

"Eight years old," she began, voice splintering into dendritic cracks. The bull-headed ant abandoned its ankle expedition as Sarah's pulse hit 112 bpm - threshold for mammalian prey signatures. Above, a nuthatch froze mid-grub extraction, sensing the seismic shift in human bioelectric fields.

Lachlan's field notes wrote themselves behind clenched teeth: *Subject exhibits vasoconstriction in extremities, pupil dilation mismatch between eyes...* His whisky tongue remembered the Kyoto board member who'd vapor locked describing his father's logging empire.

Sarah's French manicure found canyon-deep grooves in the stone. "Dusk came needle-fast," she whispered. Hemlock saplings along the clearing edge released a protective aerosol of alpha-pinene, mistaking her trauma chemistry for bark beetle invasion.

Kenji's herb pouch leaked linalool across the circle, his grandfather's voice murmuring through crushed leaves: *When the heart races, find what's rooted.* Aisha's scarf absorbed panic pheromones, its Kampala jasmine threads swelling with the effort.

"The rangers' flashlights..." Sarah's hyoid bone jerked like a hooked trout. Sixteen meters northeast, a black vine snake mirrored the motion in reverse, constricting memories of its own forest floor abandonment.

Lachlan's flask burned reproach against his femur. He'd watched doctoral candidates present peer-reviewed breakdowns with less physiological carnage. But when Sarah's left iris dilated beyond 6mm - Tokyo all over again - the moss intervened.

Plagiomnium undulatum crept over her ankles, its velvety gametophytes pumping out GABA analogs. Five species of springtail began dismantling fallen fear molecules. The forest, it seemed, remembered protocols older than ranger manuals.

As Sarah passed the stone, its glacial scars warming under Kenji's herbalist palms, the clearing exhaled twenty-three years worth of trapped frost. Somewhere beyond the tree line, phantom flashlights winked out.

The stone bloomed warmth in Kenji's palms, its Cretaceous minerals reacting to the 0.3ml of nerol oil secreted by his grandfather's herb pouch seams. Golden morning light hit the linen bundle at 57°, igniting topnotes of Edo-era pharmacies and Showa-period sweat.

"Yama-budo," he announced, unknotting indigo-dyed cloth with ritual precision. A pressed vine leaf emerged - June 1999 vintage, its serrated edges still humming with the tonal pitch of a seven-year-old's laughter.

Lachlan's nostrils flared in professional appraisal: *Akebia quinata, cardiac glycoside concentration optimal in specimen...* His pen died mid-thought, electrocuted by Kenji's sudden grin - grandfather's dentures flash in autumn woods.

The herb walk unfolded through finger braille. Kenji's thumbnail traced ulcerwort trichomes ("Count seven per mm² for fever reduction"), callus ridges catching on memories of a hand twice his size guiding the motion. Aisha's jasmine metabolites tangled with drying hagi flowers, their volatile organics debating Kampala versus Kyoto drying techniques.

"Corporate pharmacies..." Kenji's laugh lines inverted as a pharmaceutical packet fell from his satchel - blister packs mocking his kanji-labeled muslin bags. The forest countered with a downpour of Zelkova samaras, their papery wings rewriting dosage instructions in air current shorthand.

When Kenji demonstrated grandfather's arthritis balm technique, the clearing's humidity cooperated - 78% RH plumping cadaverous chickweed back to medicinal juiciness. Hana's charcoal stick betrayed her, sketching absently in margins: old man hands cradling dogwood bark.

The stone passed fungal custody - Kenji's *Saccharomyces cerevisiae* colonies handshaking with Hana's graphite microbiome. Somewhere beyond the cedars, a telephone-pole fungi absorbed decades of herbal wisdom through its concrete diet. Lachlan's flask approved via tarnished smirk.

The stone weighed like a curator's rejection letter in Hana's grip, her thumbnail blackened with charcoal that predated gallery white cubes. Her Moleskine breathed its last humid breath, pages curling into sea anemone shapes that mocked Tokyo's climate-controlled vitrines.

"Art Basel Hong Kong 2022," she began, voice dust-dry as compressed graphite. A speckled slug crossed her toe, trailing mucus that mirrored the sheen on her last lacquered sculpture. The forest leaned in - squirrel cache maps overwriting Hana's abandoned grid paper.

Lachlan noted the 0.7mm tremor in her dominant hand - residual damage from three consecutive nights rendering steel wool clouds under LED interrogation. A cicada shell crunched under her shifting knee, its abdominal segments echoing the ribbed vents of her Chelsea studio's HVAC system.

"Critics praised my 'urban sterility series'." Her laugh flaked like bad gesso. The sketchpad bled willow charcoal memories - twelve years old, burning branches in grandfather's kiln to make Honmonji Temple offering sticks.

A sudden downpour of maple keys jammed her

pause. Hana's fingers moved autonomously, capturing the aerodynamic spin that had once fascinated aerospace engineers. The lines thickened uncontrollably, her Rotring pen's ghost screaming at the organic heresy.

Kenji's mint leaves wilted in solidarity as she described her Shibuya apartment - sealed windows preserving emptiness at 21°C, the potted *Ficus benjamina*'s silent judgment. The stone passed through a beam of forest light that had evaded 3000K gallery spots for centuries, its warmth conducting through Aisha's jasmine oil fingerprints directly into Hana's median nerve.

When a woodlouse navigated her sketch's margins, Hana didn't flick it away but noted how its segmented armor outclassed her best metallic pigments. The forest had drafted its review in arthropod hieroglyphs.

The stone dripped jasmine hydrosol onto Aisha's lap, her scarf's silk proteins slowly releasing 2003 courtyard dew points. She inhaled the mirage - grandmother's cracked clay ollas sweating more faithfully than Tokyo's titanium taps.

"We had seven fountains," she began, fingers mapping hydraulic patterns in air. Lachlan's inner zoologist logged the motion - identical to Jordanian desert foxes tracing underground rivers through paw tremors.

Kenji's herb pouch sneezed mint at her description of za'atar hedges. The corporate warrior's Prada mules dug graves for themselves in loam, their thermoplastic soles rejecting the memory of Damascus rose petals crushed en route to French perfumeries.

"Condominium board banned balcony planters." Aisha's laugh vibrated at the frequency of snapped olive saplings. The stone warmed to blood heat, conducting visions of her clandestine avocado pit nursery glowing under 4000K bathroom lighting.

A carpenter bee mistook her scarf for cerumen, depositing pollen bribes against Egyptian cotton's embargo. Lachlan noted the exact moment Aisha's Achilles tendon remembered mud - 4:32PM, solar angle triggering cellular memory of monsoon irrigation channels.

When she described smuggling gardenia clippings through Dubai customs, the clearing's ferns released spores in solidarity. Hana's charcoal stick surrendered completely, snapping to sketch root systems that breached concrete fantasies.

As the stone passed westward, it carried topnotes of stolen topsoil and three generations of women's palm lines mapped onto watering can handles. The taniwha flask approved through tarnish patterns only ancestral gardeners could parse.

The stone returned as accusatory relic, its ammonite spirals dissecting Lachlan's career into fossil layers. He rotated it once for each rejected paper - nineteen revolutions aligning with Hiroshi's bamboo groove count.

"Published seven papers on *Cryptomeria japonica*," he began, thumbnail scoring the stone's Jurassic growth bands. The clearing inhaled - katydids silencing for the man who'd cataloged their chitin microstructure but missed the symphony.

Kyoto's winter chill resurrected in his sacrum - 2014 fieldwork, thermocouple probes violating a cedar's frost-heave rhythm. The tree's retaliation had come as dendrochronological roast: 1672 fire scars pulsing in time with his mother's final EKG flatline.

Sarah's ruined blouse rustled a standing ovation as he described sabotaging his own traps. Kenji's grandfather's watch approved via radioactive glow - radium dial hands embracing after eighty years of manufactured separation.

When Lachlan revealed the flask's new contents ("Distilled dawn transpiration from this clearing"), Hana's charcoal stick finally achieved flight - a dragonfly deposition system outperforming gallery installation budgets.

The group's palms met earth in fungal matrimony, ringed by Lachlan's discarded pager still buzzing with dean's ultimatums. Mycelia threaded through cuticles, converting LinkedIn anxieties into chanterelle promises.

As twilight credentialed them all honorary myrmecologists, the stones began their slow work of forgetting names. Somewhere beyond the forest, a university website updated its faculty page - error 404 rising like mayfly wings where Lachlan's CV once nested.

The Forest's True Treasure

Afternoon light struck the cedar colonnade at 57.3 degrees, fracturing gold across Lachlan's path like a dendrochronologist's puzzle. His thumb rubbed the satchel's worn whale clasp— Christchurch conference dust still embedded in its jade eye—as twenty-three moss-capped stones whispered directions their GPS couldn't comprehend. The clearing unfolded its secrets in layers: first the cinnamon tang of decaying Tsuga needles, then the fractal geometry of maidenhair fern shadows, finally the collective intake of breath as five pairs of urbanized lungs met air unsullied by combustion engines.

Sarah's REI tent poles clicked with military precision, her Stanford ring flashing semaphore against the gloom. "Site B secured," she announced to nobody, driving a titanium stake through loam that had nourished trees when her Ivy League alma mater was still a marsh. The collapsed backpack spat out gear sorted by REI product codes—a waterproof sack labeled FORAGE clinging stubbornly to its factory creases. When a maple key helicoptered into her part-line, she paused just long enough to classify its descent rate before tucking it behind her ear like a woodland memo.

Thirty paces northwest, Kenji's nose hovered three centimeters above a lichen-crusted log. "*Lactarius volemus*," he murmured, grandfather's hand lens swinging pendulum-like from its rawhide cord. The specimen's apricot aroma triggered memories of bento boxes in Sendai cedar groves—sun-warm rice, mother's warning finger tapping venomous *Galerina* lookalikes. His field knife hesitated at the mushroom's base, blade edge catching seven overlapping spore patterns that whispered warnings about corporate biohacking ventures.

Hana's charcoal stick rebelled against the clearing's chaos, its sharp tip skating across paper made from trees that never knew concrete. The cedar before her spread roots like varicose veins, bark ridges forming faces that mocked her gallery contracts. "Commission guidelines require perspective lines," she reminded the sketchpad, but her wrist disobeyed, capturing instead the exact angle where a lightning scar dissolved into woodpecker apartments. When the charcoal snapped, she pressed the jagged edge into paper grain until cellulose bled shadows matching the forest floor's braille.

Aisha's silk scarf became a reliquary for chlorophyll saints—sassafras leaves whispering Kampala monsoons, ginkgo fans fanning memories of grandmother's medicinal teas. Her once-manicured nail traced a white oak vein's branching logic, corporate acquisition strategies crumbling before xylem's ancient flow. "You'd thrive in container gardens," she assured a spicebush seedling, its leaves already compiling rebuttals to high-rise HVAC systems.

"Notice the Tsuga's apical dominance," Lachlan called, voice softening as a fawn's ear flickered through bracken. His lecture on terminal buds died mid-syllable—the yearling's wobble-kneed curiosity transcending arboricultural jargon. Somewhere behind ocular orbits hardened by thirty-seven peer reviews, a fourteen-year-old self stirred, pressing against the Toyota's rear window to count migrating kāmahi flowers.

As shadows stretched their dendritic arms

across the clearing, Lachlan's flask found itself repurposed as a magnifier for Aisha's leaf collection. "See the trichome patterns?" he asked, Islay malt distorting through curved glass into amber rivers. "Same defense mechanism as Ugandan acacias." Sarah's tent stake hit something stone-solid and pre-Meiji, her corporate timbre cracking as she unearthed a moss-crusted kogo incense vessel. Kenji's mycological harvest expanded to include chanterelle lookalikes and the exact mushroom that poisoned Emperor Go-Toba's favorite concubine.

Dusk arrived as avian shift change—scolding jays surrendering to barred owl interrogations, last cedar waxwings drunken on fermented pyracantha berries. Hana's sketchbook absorbed twilight through paper pores, transforming into something that might finally please both gallery owners and wood ant colonies. Aisha's scarf, now a mosaic of deciduous martyrs, fluttered semaphore between pines as the first cricket tuned its wings to C-sharp minor. Lachlan's satchel slumped against nurse log, its leather slowly remembering how to be tree bark again.

Flames licked Sarah's last corporate spreadsheet to ash, its waterproof paper curling like the arthritic fingers of CFOs she'd never appease. The firepit became a Rorschach altar—Hana's crooked log teepee vomiting sparks that died inches from Aisha's Kampala-scented hair. Kenji fed the blaze with monastic precision, each twig a medicinal offering: juniper for purification, magnolia leaves for fractured attention spans, pine resin for the ghost of his grandfather's TB-ravaged lungs.

The freeze-dried meals protested their resurrection, Mountain House beef stroganoff yielding to Aisha's foraged wood sorrel and chanterelles still sweating Hiroshi's bamboo grove dew. Sarah's titanium spork hovered over the communal pot, her hypothalamus lighting up at flavors no boardroom caterer could replicate—the exact umami note of *Lactarius* mushrooms that once fueled samurai midnight marches. Across the flames, Hana's jaw unclenched in millimeter increments, tendon by tendon, as roasted burdock root resurrected memories of charcoal pencils stolen from a Sendai stationary shop.

When Lachlan's flask first breached the

firelight, its taniwha engraving writhed in the heat shimmer. The whiskey's journey began with Sarah—a perfunctory sip that became three, her CEO veneer dissolving as Lagavulin's peat smoke met Tsuga resin lingering in her sinuses. Kenji's lips moved in silent apology to grandfather's sobriety oaths before the liquor hit his ulcerated stomach lining with the grace of Kōyasan monks breaking fast.

"Noticed this today," Sarah began, shoulders rolling through a range of motion her physical therapist had billed in 15-minute increments. "Took a Zoom call under white pine. Realized I wasn't...counting milliseconds till the next agenda item." A firefly alighted on her spreadsheet-scarred index finger, its abdomen pulsing like a cursor begging forgiveness.

Kenji's demonstration started with Meiji-era breathing ratios but collapsed into wheezing laughter when an owl hooted the Jingle Bells melody. "Asthma attack at Yakushima research station," he gasped between inhalations of air so crisp it could etch glass. "Old-growth sugi resins worked better than Albuterol." The group's exhales synchronized—eighteen months of trapped smog departing in unison.

Hana's sketchbook fell open to a cedar rendered in emergency room lighting. "My 'ally' dropped a branch on my tent week one," she confessed, charcoal smudges mimicking the bruise's yellow-green decay. The fire popped its critique as she revealed today's pages—a root system mirroring her own vascular network, corporate coffee stains transformed into fungal halos.

Aisha's braids swung like pendulum bobs counting down to revelation. "Seventy-three empty rooftops," she stated, fingers dancing with borrowed firelight. "Each could host a forest bathing podium." The word tasted foreign—a Kampala childhood term for grandmother's medicinal porch. Above, the Milky Way etched equations even Sarah's algorithms couldn't parse.

Lachlan let the silence swell, flask draining as Orion's belt aligned with the firepit stones. "Found three new fungal hybrids last month," he began, voice fraying like overused climbing rope. "None publishable." The admission hung heavier than his canceled keynote address. "But this—" his palm upturned to catch falling maple samara "—this collaboration between wing geometry and convective lift? This is the methodology we've been missing."

106

Embers sketched mortality timelines across Sarah's upturned palms, each wrinkle briefly illuminated like quarterly reports she'd once laminated for immortality. The fire's death rattle sent sparks spiraling into Hana's overturned sketchbook—a Moleskine requiem burning with the particular stench of creative compromise. Somewhere beyond the ring of stones, Tokyo's light pollution lost its grip on the atmosphere, allowing Antares to pierce through with the exact red of Aisha's childhood nail polish.

"I sold my Birkin for forest therapy certification," Sarah announced to the Pleiades, fingers working the clasp of a platinum necklace that had strangled more ideas than corporate bylaws. The chain slithered into the ashes, its sapphire pendant winking like the last server light in a data center shutdown. Her abandoned phone buzzed faintly underground, its aluminum skeleton slowly remembering ore formed during the Great Oxidation Event.

Kenji poured chrysanthemum tea through grandfather's cracked infuser, steam curling into the exact shape of his abandoned pharmaceutical sales targets. "Seven breaths per morning," he stated, wrist tilting to align with Polaris. "Not quarterly profits." The leaves settled into a sediment map of Mount Zaō's last eruption—a topography his ancestors would have recognized as divine tea reading.

Hana's arm swept through the smoke like an exorcism, depositing twelve pounds of urban sketches into the pyre. "Commissions can choke," she declared as flaming ginkgo leaves rose like phoenixes from the paper's grain. The new charcoal stick she pulled from ashes still pulsed with the heartbeat of whatever maple had died to birth it.

Aisha's fingers danced through moonlit GIS coordinates, her scarf's jasmine threads weaving Tokyo's concrete gaps into grandmother's folk songs. "Playground here," she stabbed air where a pachinko parlor blighted city maps. "Community garden here," palm slapping space inhabited by a love hotel's neon despair. Above, the Milky Way mirrored Kampala's rainy season constellation maps with unsettling precision.

When the final log collapsed into carbonized regret, Lachlan remained guard over glowing remnants, his flask now filled with cedar infusion from Hiroshi's last grove. The

taniwha's scales had shifted under heat stress—
its jade eyes now mirroring the exact moss-
flecked amber of Sarah's abandoned pendant.
Somewhere beyond the tents, a sapling cracked
its nursery pot confines, roots whispering
through volcanic soil towards Sarah's buried
sapphire—the forest's newest mycorrhizal
collaborator.

The Skeptic's Challenge

The rental sedan's door thunk shut with laboratory precision, its metallic echo scarring the forest's morning hush. Dr. Evelyn Blackwood's leather portfolio hissed against raw silk blouse as she surveyed the gaggle of urban refugees contaminating the trailhead. Twelve meters east, Lachlan McGregor's weathered palm cradled a thermos emitting whiskey-tinged steam, his smile crinkling beard hairs that held last week's cedar resin like insect specimens in amber.

"Dr. Blackwood." His boots compressed three mushroom species during the approach—Shiitake, nameko, and an *Amanita* guessing game. "Your emails undersold the..." The sentence died as her Louboutin sank into loam, heel gulped whole by soil pH-balanced to dissolve corporate pretension.

Sarah's fingers betrayed her first—tremors vibrating collection vials into wind chime discordance. She cataloged Blackwood's armor: Burberry trench repelling mist, Ferragamo crossbody digesting thirty years of forest therapy meta-analyses. Kenji's thumb polished grandfather's spectacles into defensive shields, the motion activating muscle memory from defending thesis methodologies to sneering reviewers.

"The cortisol sampling lacks proper controls." Blackwood's Montblanc stabbed air where Hiroshi's bamboo wind chimes once translated typhoon warnings. "Your phytoncide exposure metrics resemble..." A maple key intervened, kamikaze-diving into the precise gray strand maintaining her chignon's martial order.

Lachlan produced vials from his whiskey-scented satchel, morning light fracturing through glass into Sarah's palms. "Salivettes for science." His grin widened as a *Lasius japonicus* battalion scaled Blackwood's patent leather portfolio, carrying aphid eggs past her ANOVA tables. "We'll chart what eludes quantification."

Aisha's braids swept fern data sheets into temporary burial. "In Uganda, we measure mango yields by bark thickness." Her Kampala cadence softened Blackwood's flinch at "anecdotal evidence." The psychologist's clipboard angled defensively—a Spartan shield against organic heresy.

When Lachlan described midnight epiphanies beneath radioactive cedars, Blackwood's pen froze mid-scribble. Her sleeve snagged on bark oozing Cretaceous memories, amber droplets preserving damning dendrological evidence across Chanel sleeve guards. The forest inhaled—thirty-seven fungal species digesting skepticism into fertile humus.

Sarah's vial became a prism scattering Corporate Woman into wavelengths the woods could parse. Somewhere beyond the parking lot's dying asphalt, seven crows reshuffled power lines into a staff only Hiroshi could read.

Blackwood's stopwatch beeped its fifth interval as Sarah choked on air suddenly thick with decaying hemlock and desperation. The psychologist's UV-protected clipboard shed water like mallard feathers, repelling maple samaras armed with aerodynamic contempt.

"Focus on the stream's arrhythmia," Lachlan urged, knee-deep in metaphors and *Hydrangea serrata*. His thumb circled clockwise—a gesture Hiroshi once used to quiet argumentative grad students. Sarah's Apple Watch vibrated treasonous encouragement as the water reshaped her "urgent" into "ripples."

Hana's charcoal stick snapped, its jagged edge mirroring the cedar's lightning scar. "You want perspective lines?" she challenged the forest, smearing humus across paper until corporate commissions dissolved into mycelial truth.

Blackwood's pedometer choked on inconsistent terrain. Her Ferragamo sole met cypress knee with a crack louder than p-values hitting zero. "Statistical outliers," she muttered, but her voice wavered as Kenji's cedar released a pollen cloud that bypassed her N95 mask to deliver memories of childhood tree forts.

"Your methodology assumes linear causation," Blackwood accused, but the words emerged softer, filtered through phytoncides that remembered when peer review meant elders tasting bark for winter predictions.

Golden hour found Blackwood's tablet screen overrun with pollen armies, each grain a taunting exclamation point against her ANOVA tables. Kenji hovered like a samurai pharmacist, grandfather's asthma graphs overlapping modern cytokine curves in damning harmony.

"Your T-cell readings resemble Grandfather's herb logs," he offered, *Armillaria* sprouting from his abandoned inhaler. Sarah's laughter shook loose data points that Hana captured with charcoal—stress metrics reborn as *Betula* shadow puppets.

The forest celebrated its invasion of science. Slime mold etched Fibonacci critiques across consent forms. A *Geotrupes* battalion dragged Blackwood's voice recorder into pagan communion. When she reached to intervene, *Cryptomeria* resin stitched temporary fingerprints to latex.

"Correlation...requires replication," Blackwood choked, throat tight with Hiroshi's phytoncides. Her gloveless hand brushed *Neolentinus suffrutescens*, its bioluminescence outshining LCD displays.

Lachlan materialized with beetle-annotated journals. "Happatsu Yakushi's monks measured enlightenment through lichen growth." His thumb rested where Blackwood's pulse fluttered like netted wren.

The stolen Tsuga cone burned her blazer pocket with cellular truths. As rental car sensors blipped rebuke, a single breath—five seconds over recommended duration—stole *Chamaecyparis* volatile organics she'd later call "contaminants" in drafts never published.

Aisha's honey jar waited passenger-side, its comb geometry echoing the leaf mandala already photosynthesizing in Blackwood's notes. Somewhere beyond the parking lot's dying asphalt, seven crows reshuffled power lines into a staff even Cornell couldn't parse.

Lost in Doubt

The manila envelopes crackled like alien bark in Lachlan's grip, their corners dented from riding shotgun with Hiroshi's bamboo charcoal samples. Morning mist curled around his wrists, recoiling from the documents' formaldehyde reek. Behind him, the trailhead cedars stood motionless - not the usual attentive sentinels, but bored security guards checking nature's wristwatch.

Kenji's sneeze detonated prematurely. "Is that—?" he began, knuckles whitening around a handkerchief embroidered with his grandfather's asthma clinic logo. Lachlan's thumbnail slit the envelope's gummy seal, releasing a waft of toner fumes that made Aisha's jasmine perfume retreat behind her collarbones.

"Phytoncide exposure..." Lachlan's voice caught on the Latinate syllables. The stamp bled through the paper's grain - INCONCLUSIVE in bureaucrat red, consuming Sarah's cortisol graphs like kudzu over a shrine gate. Hana's charcoal stick snapped against her sketchbook spine, graphite dust snowing across a half-finished rendering of the forest's vascular system.

The maples withheld their usual commentary. No samaras helicoptered into Sarah's immaculate blowout; no woodpeckers provided percussive emphasis. Even Lachlan's trusty flask sat heavy in his satchel, its taniwha engraving tarnished by sweat from his 4AM parking lot rereading.

Kenji's finger hovered over a p-value. "0.067. That's... almost significant?" His laugh unspooled like a snapped guywire, startling a cabbage white butterfly from his shoulder. The insect's erratic flight pattern mapped the group's disintegrating confidence.

Aisha's phone buzzed against quartz bedrock, its screen casting LED shame across lichen colonies. She thumbnailed the notification into oblivion. "Tokyo Urban Development Board," she translated for the unmoving cedars. "'Vertical garden proposal... cost-prohibitive structural modifications required.'" Her Kampala childhood emerged in the vowels, softening corporate blade-strokes with equatorial humidity.

Lachlan's boot sole ground the envelope's gummy flap into volcanic soil. "Methodological limitations," he recited to a disinterested slug, "small sample size introducing Type II error potential." The words tasted of Yuki's disappointed silence after his first failed tree whispering trial - that same chalkboard residue lingering behind molars.

Hana's sketchbook pages flapped like injured cranes. "I turned down the Mori Art Museum commission for this," she told a disintegrating charcoal cedar. "They wanted sterile topiaries. I chose *authenticity*." The last word dripped enough acid to etch glass.

A sudden pressure drop silenced Sarah's data-driven rebuttals. The forest inhaled through clenched stomata, withholding its usual terpene bouquet. Somewhere beyond perception, Hiroshi's bamboo chimes hung motionless, their song trapped in the limbo between scientific rigor and arboreal truth.

Kenji's allergy meds chose the cedar's base camp to mutate into biochemical traitors. His fingers swelled around the amber bottle - "Immune Harmony Blend" kanji strokes blurring behind condensation and hives.

Grandfather's spectacles slid down his sebum-slick nose as he squinted at ingredients that now read like betrayal: reishi mushroom, Japanese mugwort, and what the optimistic label called "ancient sugi resilience extract."

The forest retaliated in airstrikes of pollen. Lachlan watched a birch catkin explode its payload directly into Kenji's orbital zone, the golden particulate adhering to moisturizer and despair. "Maybe it's psychosomatic," he offered weakly, flask unscrewed with his non-charred hand. The whiskey's peat smoke curdled mid-air, failing to mask Kenji's sneeze-propelled snot globule hitting a spider's dewdrop chandelier.

Twenty paces northwest, Hana's charcoal enacted revenge for last night's disparaging Yelp review. Each stroke on the "100% Recycled!" sketchbook disintegrated into graphite shrapnel, the paper's tooth grabbing her lines like a jealous lover. "It was supposed to *flow*," she told a disinterested slug, thumbnail gouging the cedar's shadow into something resembling corporate flowcharts. Her commissioner's voice haunted the margins: "More structure, Ms. Nakamura. Clients need recognizability."

Aisha's phone screen spiderwebbed its grief across an email attachment titled "Structural Integrity Concerns.pdf." The cracks bent municipal approval stamps into avant-garde constellations, almost beautiful enough to distract from twelve weeks of terraced herb garden plans being composted. "They suggested plastic topiaries," she informed a mycelial network unimpressed by CAD renderings. "UV-resistant polyethylene. Maintenance-free."

The forest deployed biological humor. A swallowtail butterfly's wing scales triggered Kenji's fourth sneezing fit, its polka dots swimming in his tear-duct overflow. Lachlan's standard bark texture exercise went mutagenic - the hinoki's grooves suddenly mimicking Sarah's cortisol graphs under electron microscopy. Even the whiskey betrayed him, its usual vanilla undertones replaced by the tinny aftertaste of peer-reviewed failure.

Slime mold oozed across Hana's dropped eraser, its plasmodial veins diagramming a more compelling forest portrait than her trembling hand could manage. She nearly missed the notification from Mori Arts Center - "Regret to inform you" auto-translating to charcoal snaps and a bark dent that would

120

outlive them all.

By sundown, Kenji's forearms resembled a topographical map of Hokkaido, Aisha's phone battery suicided into moss, and Lachlan's flask brimmed with allergy meds dissolved in defeated single-malt. The cedars watched their retreat through resinous tears that smelled suspiciously of pyrrhic victory.

Sunlight fell through the canopy like rented stage lighting, the dapples too uniform, too obedient. Lachlan's palm met cedar bark in a handshake that left both parties embarrassed. Somewhere beyond the clearing's cruel proscenium arch, a jay coughed its disapproval.

"Focus on the... the textural gradients," he recited, thumb finding the exact knot where Yuki's laughter once vibrated through xylem. The wood felt neutered beneath his touch - no thrum of ascending sap, no whisper of century-old gossip. His whiskey flask left a tarnished halo on the roots, its taniwha's jade eyes milky with cataracts.

The group performed their roles through muscle memory. Kenji's inhaler punctuated meditation counts in 4/4 time, pharmaceutical mist mingling with missing phytoncides. Hana traced concentric circles without lifting charcoal from paper, creating a carbon black hole that swallowed three pages. Aisha's cracked phone cast LED runes across maple roots, her Kampala soil amendments proposal now composting in municipal servers.

The forest withheld commentary. No ants marched across open journals to correct data. No woodpeckers drummed peer reviews. Even the air stagnated like conference hall HVAC exhaust, none of cedar's usual cinnamon rebuttals to human folly.

When the leaf descended, it fell with insulting precision - a perfect maple samara spinning clockwise against all aerodynamic logic. It landed equidistant from all shoes, the veins spelling "INCONCLUSIVE" in chlorophyll braille. Lachlan counted seven aborted movements - Hana's wrist twitch, Aisha's inhaled breath, Kenji's phalangeal tremor - before collective resignation iced their muscles.

His flask's final gulp tasted of aquarium water and printer toner. Somewhere beyond the clearing, Hiroshi's bamboo chimes remained motionless, their silence the only peer review that mattered now. The cedars watched through narrowed growth rings as the group dispersed, their footsteps erasing nothing, their doubts fertilizing everything.

Lachlan's Solitary Sojourn

The leather satchel slumped against the tent canvas like a reproachful colleague, its whalebone clasp digging crescent moons into a resignation letter gone stiff with dew. Lachlan's thumb found the cedar resin sealant oozing through his pocket's lining - seven days since Yuki pressed it there, thirteen hours since the peer review board declared it 'statistically insignificant.' He unzipped the main compartment with surgeon's care, vials of phytoncide samples clinking accusation from their foam sarcophagus. Three protein bars fell like cadavers into his palm, their foil wrappers reflecting the exact metallic gray of Hiroshi's last stormcloud prediction.

The whiskey flask rolled into view, its taniwha's jade eyes crusted with Nikkō hot spring minerals. He pressed the cool metal to his jugular before remembering the hoarse confession he'd poured into a Kyoto storm drain - twelve-year Lagavulin mixing with sacred runoff while salarymen vomited karaoke lyrics uphill. His field journal stuck to itself when opened, pages fused by sap wept from a lightning-struck pine during their failed July measurements. A pressed frond of *Selaginella helvetica* crumbled between observation notes, its resurrection promise mocking the graphs' flatlined data.

Pen met paper where Hiroshi's trail map merged with Blackwood's rejection letter. The hybrid document buckled under first strokes, fibers rejecting bic ballpoint ink in favor of bloodroot pigment he'd used to mark sacred cedars. An orb weaver descended on dragline silk, abdomen patterning the exact hexadecimal brown of his university's letterhead. He wrote "Gone to verify" before scratching it into dendrite shapes, the nib catching on wood pulp imperfections that spelled *failure* in Dutch elm disease patterns.

Nightfall found him hip-deep in a stream that erased days. His boots hung from a persimmon sapling like executed traitors, soles turned up to reveal Sarah's cortisol maps dissolving in the current. Crayfish navigated his submerged ankles with military precision, claws snapping at the digital watch face still displaying

Blackwood's appointment reminder. A mayfly landed on the 02:47 readout, its ephemeral wings echoing the lifespan of their T-cell activation theories.

The clearing opened its arms at moon zenith. Lachlan's hatchet bounced off ironwood, vibrations traveling through blisters formed during the bow drill's mockery. His third match died in a breath that carried Yuki's favorite reproach - *Western hurry makes weak fire* - before flame finally took purchase in birch bark scrolls. The tarp sagged between twin oaks like a failed lung, collecting darkness instead of rain. He counted seven collapsing attempts before letting guy wires tangle like synaptic misfires.

By the fire's false dawn, his left palm mapped every ridge of the tenure denial letter through its ashes. Embers arranged themselves into Blackwood's margin notes - *methodologically unsound* glowing brightest in iron-rich bark. When the last cedar log cracked its vertebrae, the sound mirrored the snap of Hana's charcoal stick across her abandoned commission contract. His tongue found the ulcer where Kenji's allergy pills had lodged during that final disastrous data review, bitterness outlasting even the forest's most astringent mosses.

126

Dawn arrived as a thief, light fingers extracting night's coins from cedar bark vaults. Lachlan's boot soles registered the exact moment forest became temple - volcanic grit transmuting to nave stones beneath feet still patterned with conference hall carpet fibers. The compass needle spun like a disgraced academic avoiding eye contact, its north now aligned with the cedar's heartwood magnetic pull. He stepped over a fallen birch wearing Hiroshi's face in its decay patterns, purification sachet crumbs leaving anaphylactic trails for doubting spirits.

Bark met palm with courtroom formality. Lachlan's fingertips mapped cambium ridges that outnumbered Blackwood's citation indices, each groove a peer review surviving centuries of beetle audits. His forehead pressed the trunk's northwest face where Yuki once pinned a haiku to the kami, lignin swallowing syllables of her final admonishment - *measure less, mourn less*. Rain's first warning shot hit a holly leaf tuned to middle C, its vibration travelling sapwood channels to thrum against his left tibia.

Resin oozed over his watch crystal, amber time capsule preserving a mosquito that dined on postdoc blood. He counted breaths through clenched molars: thirty-seven (Sarah's cortisol baseline), sixty-two (Hana's rejected gallery proposals), eighty-nine (the exact number of fungal hybrids dismissed as "anecdotal"). Rain escalated its assault, each drop exploding against cedar scales to release mirages - Blackwood's Montblanc stabbing his grant proposals, Kenji's grandfather dissolving into spore clouds, Aisha's skyscraper gardens collapsing into dandelion clocks.

At ninety-three breaths, his occipital lobe fired tenure denial letters across dendrite branches. Peer review comments bored through cambium in woodpecker staccato, their rhythm syncopating with the cedar's ultrasonic screams. Then - a rogue memory synapse: mother's hands polishing a hope chest's cedar lining, his four-year-old cheek pressed against wood that smelled of forever. Rain found his optic nerves, dissolving impact factors into the fractal beauty of xylem cross-sections.

The cedar's pulse emerged as subsonic AUM. One hundred eight exhalations etched themselves into growth rings as his cerebellum decoded seven rain dialects - sleet's staccato, drizzle's rubato, mist's legato. When the downpour relented, his retinas held afterimages of Hiroshi's bamboo chimes translating neutron scattering patterns into shakuhachi meditations. The taniwha flask, forgotten against a knee, overflowed with perfect phytoncidic tears.

Morning light fell through the canopy as divine chromatography, separating Lachlan's remaining doubts into spectra that dappled the abandoned spectrometer. His bare heel sank into sphagnum moss tuned to E-flat, its vibrations rewriting Blackwood's footnotes beneath layers of ancestral peat. The forest floor issued its syllabus through plantar nerves - feather moss (Unit 1: Ephemeral Taxonomies), stair-step moss (Module 3: Mycorrhizal Ethics), and the treacherous slick of *Marchantia polymorpha* (Final Exam: Surrender).

Hands cupped behind ears caught spider silk orchest rations, draglines humming with prey alerts that translated to "see/feel/breathe." A pileated woodpecker's critique of dying birch - three staccato, two flourish - mirrored his department chair's punctuation during that disastrous tenure review. But here, the downy's morse code spelled "mercy," and the sapsucker's arrhythmia became anthems for

Hana's rejected installations.

Wineberries burst against his molars with the exact acidity of Blackwood's peer review. Morels, sautéed in a tin cup over Hiroshi's ghost fire, synthesized Yuki's laughter with tenure denial notices into umami absolution. He spat dandelion latex onto granite, its bitterness diffusing into forest hum that whispered *enough*.

The journal's pages warped into bark parchment. Lachlan's thumb smeared oak gall ink across a sketch merging cedar rings with Kenji's lung capacity charts. Beetle frass pigment spelled margins in mycelial script: *Impact factor = photosynthesis rate ÷ human hubris*. When barred owls began their nocturnal audit, he plucked a primary feather from moonlit duff, its vanes cutting truer than any institutional letterhead.

Dawn found him singing to the cedar in forgotten Māori vowels learned from his father's funeral program. The taniwha flask, refilled with hollyhock dew and woodpecker breath, sloshed confirmation against his hip. His last journal entry sealed in fireweed silk read: "Tenure grows where datasets decay - please forward all correspondence to the mycelium network." The forest's exit exam required only that he leave the compass nailed to a paper birch with his last stainless steel hypothesis, its needle quivering between lost and found.

Renewal Through Roots

The trail's volcanic grit surrendered to moss-capped limestone where clearing began, Lachlan's boot sole registering the exact moment solitude became communion. Morning light struck his whiskey flask through cedar boughs, projecting taniwha shadow-puppets across Sarah's shoulder blades as she turned— her posture no longer a steel rod of corporate readiness, but the supple curve of mountain bamboo after typhoon season.

Kenji emerged from fern shadows sneezing pentatonic scale, inhaler pocketed beneath grandfather's herb pouch. Hana's fingers worried a charcoal nub against sketchbook seams, leaving Rorschach smudges that mirrored bark patterns overhead. Only Aisha stood motionless, Kampala-born nostrils flaring as urban perfume surrendered to loam's fungal algebra.

They converged in silence perfected through

forest apprenticeships—Sarah's Burberry sleeve absorbing cedar resins from Lachlan's embrace, Kenji's asthma rattle muted against his collarbone, Hana's graphite fingerprints transferring phantom maples to his field jacket. When Aisha pressed her forehead to his whiskey-scented sternum, the jasmine in her braids debated mycorrhizal truths with last night's rain trapped in his beard.

"The cedars..." Lachlan's thumb found the cracked whalebone clasp of his satchel, releasing pressed specimens that floated downward like arboreal confetti. "They measure in growth rings, not impact factors." His palm upturned revealed a crescent of dried phloem where bark had bonded with skin for seventy-two uninterrupted hours.

Sarah's knuckle brushed the imprint. "Your cortisol graphs..."

"...Lie quieter now." He nodded to a velvet mite ascending her blazer's warped pinstripes. "The trees keep different ledgers."

Kenji's sneeze dissected the silence. "108 breaths—grandfather counted these during bronchial attacks." His fingernail tapped the flask's engraved numbers. "Coincidence?"

"Synchronicity," Lachlan corrected, watching Hana sketch the mite's path. Her charcoal snapped, unleashing a graphite meteor that cratered near Aisha's mud-caked mule.

"The willow by Nagara River," Hana murmured, "it sketched itself through my window each monsoon." Her boot scuffed evidence of last week's self-doubt into humus.

Aisha extracted a park map from her silk layers—ink bleeding across proposed garden plots into Rorschach wetlands. "There's a ginkgo near Sendagaya Station," she offered, tear salts fixing the coordinates permanently. "Its roots chew through concrete like old bones."

Lachlan's flask arced sunlight into their midst. "Find your taniwha. Not subjects—allies." The whiskey's peat smoke sketched possibilities in air: Sarah's pine surviving fault lines, Kenji's elm hosting pharmacopoeias in its skirts, Hana's willow translating wind into brushstrokes, Aisha's ginkgo straddling subway vents.

As cicadas resumed their quantum calculations, the forest sighed through seven hundred stomata. Sarah's stiletto—last bastion of urban armor—sank reverently into nurse log pulp.

Sunlight fractured across the outcrop in honeycomb cells, each hexagonal pool a test chamber for Sarah's rediscovered humility. Her stiletto hesitated where granite met pioneer moss—the pine above oozing resin stalactites that mirrored conference room clock drips. Pressing palms to fissured bark, she cataloged survival metrics: 43% slope grade, pH 5.6, fourteen beetle boreholes...

"Storm rings," Lachlan murmured, appearing as shadow puppetry through needle clusters. "This one survived the '98 eruptions." His thumbnail bisected a dark growth band, releasing terpene tears that gummed Sarah's abandoned corporate ID to the trunk.

Three switchbacks downhill, Kenji's nasal inhalations became herbal liturgy. The elm's buttress roots cradled a rebel pharmacy: mugwort violating asphalt seams, dandelions synthesizing cortisone, chickweed mocking his pharmaceutical spreadsheets. Crushing mitsuba leaves between thumb and forefinger, he resurrected grandmother's asthma tea rituals—until a sneeze scattered petals into perfect inhalation angles.

"Bless you," chuckled Lachlan from the fern

line, counting seven medicinal varieties the elm hosted in its understory skirt.

By the stream's silver tongue, Hana's willow performed arboreal puppetry—branch tips etching chiaroscuro through cheap sketchbook paper. Her wrist flick mirrored catkin pendulums until carpenter ants amended her strokes with pheromone signatures. "Collaborators," she muttered, smudging their trails into rootlet gradients.

Urban light pollution haunted Aisha's ginkgo hunt—smartphone GPS dying as steel reflections fused with fan-shaped leaves. Her Prada mule stubbed against a root cracking pavement in Matsukawa patterns. "There you are," she breathed, fingernail tracing where concrete cancer met photosynthetic resolve. The final 1% battery charge framed their union: Glass towers and chlorophyll veins in split-screen matrimony.

Lachlan's field notes grew damp with unregistered data: Sarah's pine bonding with abandoned spreadsheet fibers, Kenji's antihistamines composting under folkloric elm, Hana's willow teaching negative space through aphid migrations, Aisha's ginkgo digesting subway vibrations into growth spurts. His

136

whiskey flask, left deliberately empty, filled with absolution.

Afternoon light struck the clearing's quartz deposits at 57°, transmuting pine resin into liquid circuitry that connected their palms. Lachlan unspooled Hiroshi's moth-eaten prayer rope—108 knots corresponding to Sarah's cortisol dip, Kenji's allergy reduction, Hana's sketchpad revisions, Aisha's transit maps.

"The promise lives here," he intoned, pressing Sarah's terpene-stained thumb to Kenji's herb-crusted wrist. Their joined hands cast dendritic shadows that Hana translated into biomechanical flowcharts.

Aisha's smartphone resurrection documented pavement fissures—ginkgo roots lifting concrete like samurai armor plates. "It's teaching the sidewalk to breathe," she reported, subway tremors beneath her soles counting down to ritual hour.

Lachlan demonstrated the mudra with Yuki's ghost fingers correcting his pinky angle. "Heart to xylem, no intermediaries." Kenji's palms bloomed allergic roses against wool slacks, mirroring elm's pollen output. Sarah's earring—fresh pine amber—swung metronome circles that hypnotized a watching nuthatch.

On the 108th exhalation, Tokyo's underground railway quake reached the clearing through fungal networks. Aisha's ginkgo shivered in shared resonance, Hana's willow sketch fluttered like temple prayer board, Kenji's elm dispensed antihistamine spores, Sarah's pine hummed geologic anthems. Lachlan's abandoned pager, buried under cedar duff, dissolved its final 'Urgent' message into lichen poetry.

As shadows stretched kinship across prefectures, they dispersed—Sarah's resin earrings transmuting into pine's defensive arsenal, Kenji's elm salve crossing herbal-cultural borders, Hana's ant-collaborated sketches touring gallery sewage pipes, Aisha's smartphone photosynthesizing between subway tiles.

Lachlan remained as the forest's failed academic, whiskey flask overflowing with unmeasured phytoncide miracles. Somewhere, seven cedars adjusted their growth to shelter four new annual rings.

Confronting the Inner Critic

First light painted the cedar colonnade in foxfire gold, each needle conducting dawn's arrival through chloroplast networks older than corporate empires. Lachlan's boots sank into volcanic silt still whispering of last night's storm, the leather soles remembering thirty-seven variations of forest entry. His left palm tingled where Hiroshi's farewell grip had fused cedar resin to life lines - a cartographer's stain marking the border between academic pretense and arboreal truth.

Sarah emerged through mist wearing her Burberry trench like armor freshly lacquered, its belt cinched precisely between third and fourth rib. Beneath her designated *Pinus densiflora*, morning resin cascaded in stalactite formations that mocked the symmetrical drips of her office's abstract chandelier. When Lachlan pressed a phytoncide vial into her hand, the glass burned with residual peat smoke from his flask's all-night vigil over rejected datasets.

"Growth rings never apologize for famine years," he murmured. Sarah's neck twitched - that same involuntary spasm from age fourteen when her metronome had shattered mid-*Moonlight Sonata*, crystalline shards embedding in the Steinway's pedals. The pine's cinnamon defense chemicals now conducted through her sinuses, resurrecting the acid tang of fear-sweat on plastic piano keys.

Kenji arrived trailing competing histories - grandfather's *kinome*-scented herb pouch swinging pendulum-like against the pharmaceutical inhaler clipped to his belt. His fingers counted seven elm leaves between each labored breath, childhood asthma attacks measured in the tick-rattle of a Taishō-era pocket watch. The elm's skirt of mugwort and self-heal nodded recognition, roots still nursing the iron tang of samurai surgeons' sawbones from when these woods hosted battlefield triage.

At the willow's mourning veil, Hana's charcoal stick flayed bark textures onto paper made from pulped rejection letters. *Too controlled* hissed the RISD evaluator's voice as branches lowered a caterpillar onto her page. Its undulating body wrote liquid challenges in mucus trails, overwriting the sketched geometry of Tokyo galleries that had dismissed her "biomorphic rigidity."

Aisha's GPS died protesting as ginkgo roots cracked concrete beneath her Prada mules. "Eighteen millimeters since Tuesday," she reported, Kampala's equatorial vowels weathering the syllable edges. The sapling's roots hummed through shoe leather - not the diesel growl of Kampala-bound mango trucks, but the subsonic purr of grandmother's voice calming riots via radio. Her smartphone screen flared one last protest before dying, reflecting not her face but the old woman's smile in the fissure's dendritic spread.

When Lachlan's cedar-stained palms summoned the circle, dawn fractured through phytoncide vials to cast corporate spreadsheet grids across their chests. Sarah's first breath hitched at cinnamon revelations in her alveoli. Kenji's elbows locked mid-count as elm terpenes bypassed bronchial guards. Hana's charcoal surrendered to willow-guided strokes. And Aisha's soles resonated with the ginkgo's silent war cry against poured concrete, its roots writing new equations in the sidewalk's flesh.

"Trees keep receipts," Lachlan declared, fingers brushing cedar prayer scars Hiroshi had taught him to read like Braille. The morning ritual unfolded through imperfect geometries - Sarah's exhales syncing with sap ascent, Kenji's inhaler hissing counterpoint to Shiso photosynthesis. When the willow branch tapped Hana's wrist in approval, its leaves whispered the exact cadence of her grandmother's weaving song through paper walls.

By the third collective exhalation, the forest had rewritten their inner lexicons. Spreadsheet cells became chloroplast arrays. Profit margins dissolved into xylem mathematics. And deep in the volcanic subsoil, the cedar's roots cradled Hiroshi's bamboo timer still counting towards infinite dawns.

First light painted the cedar colonnade in foxfire gold, each needle conducting dawn's arrival through chloroplast networks older than corporate empires. Lachlan's boots sank into volcanic silt still whispering of last night's storm, the leather soles remembering thirty-seven variations of forest entry. His left palm tingled where Hiroshi's farewell grip had fused cedar resin to life lines - a cartographer's stain marking the border between academic pretense and arboreal truth.

Sarah emerged through mist wearing her Burberry trench like armor freshly lacquered, its belt cinched precisely between third and fourth rib. Beneath her designated *Pinus densiflora*, morning resin cascaded in stalactite formations that mocked the symmetrical drips of her office's abstract chandelier. When Lachlan pressed a phytoncide vial into her hand, the glass burned with residual peat smoke from his flask's all-night vigil over rejected datasets.

"Growth rings never apologize for famine years," he murmured. Sarah's neck twitched - that same involuntary spasm from age fourteen when her metronome had shattered mid-*Moonlight Sonata*, crystalline shards embedding in the Steinway's pedals. The pine's cinnamon defense chemicals now conducted through her sinuses, resurrecting the acid tang of fear-sweat on plastic piano keys.

Kenji arrived trailing competing histories - grandfather's *kinome*-scented herb pouch swinging pendulum-like against the pharmaceutical inhaler clipped to his belt. His fingers counted seven elm leaves between each labored breath, childhood asthma attacks measured in the tick-rattle of a Taishō-era pocket watch. The elm's skirt of mugwort and self-heal nodded recognition, roots still nursing the iron tang of samurai surgeons' sawbones from when these woods hosted battlefield triage.

At the willow's mourning veil, Hana's charcoal stick flayed bark textures onto paper made from pulped rejection letters. *Too controlled* hissed the RISD evaluator's voice as branches lowered a caterpillar onto her page. Its undulating body wrote liquid challenges in mucus trails, overwriting the sketched geometry of Tokyo galleries that had dismissed her "biomorphic rigidity."

Aisha's GPS died protesting as ginkgo roots cracked concrete beneath her Prada mules. "Eighteen millimeters since Tuesday," she reported, Kampala's equatorial vowels weathering the syllable edges. The sapling's roots hummed through shoe leather - not the diesel growl of Kampala-bound mango trucks, but the subsonic purr of grandmother's voice calming riots via radio. Her smartphone screen flared one last protest before dying, reflecting not her face but the old woman's smile in the fissure's dendritic spread.

When Lachlan's cedar-stained palms summoned the circle, dawn fractured through phytoncide vials to cast corporate spreadsheet grids across their chests. Sarah's first breath hitched at cinnamon revelations in her alveoli. Kenji's elbows locked mid-count as elm terpenes bypassed bronchial guards. Hana's charcoal surrendered to willow-guided strokes. And Aisha's soles resonated with the ginkgo's silent war cry against poured concrete, its roots writing new equations in the sidewalk's flesh.

"Trees keep receipts," Lachlan declared, fingers brushing cedar prayer scars Hiroshi had taught him to read like Braille. The morning ritual unfolded through imperfect geometries - Sarah's exhales syncing with sap ascent, Kenji's inhaler hissing counterpoint to Shiso photosynthesis. When the willow branch tapped Hana's wrist in approval, its leaves whispered the exact cadence of her grandmother's weaving song through paper walls.

By the third collective exhalation, the forest had rewritten their inner lexicons. Spreadsheet cells became chloroplast arrays. Profit margins dissolved into xylem mathematics. And deep in the volcanic subsoil, the cedar's roots cradled Hiroshi's bamboo timer still counting towards infinite dawns.

The pine's shadow fingers elongated across Sarah's mandala-in-progress, needled silhouettes plotting quadrants with Stock Exchange precision. Her Burberry trench lay splayed like a crime scene outline, its inner lining hosting autumn's plunder - crimson maple wings, lichen shards, and the hollow-boned remains of a fire-crawler nymph.

"Begin with what resists symmetry," Lachlan instructed, kneading a pinecone until scales fell like disgraced bar graphs. Sarah's fingers twitched phantom spreadsheet shortcuts - Ctrl+Shift+L to filter imperfections from data sets. She arranged scarlet oak leaves clockwise, their serrations aligned to 0.5mm tolerance.

An acorn disrupted the pattern, rolling diagonally across her Excel-perfect grid. Sarah's neck tendon twanged, resurrecting the ghost pain of all-nighters auditing merger proposals. Lachlan crouched, breath whisky-warm against her mandala's fault line. "Nature's CFO prefers creative accounting."

As he scattered birch catkins, Sarah's muscle memory conjured the glass-smooth finish of her corner office desk. The materials rebelled - twisted sweetgum balls refusing parallel placement, hawk moth wings collapsing under their own iridescence. When an ant battalion commandeered a pine nut tribute, their chaotic march mirrored Nasdaq's opening bell bedlam.

Lachlan produced Hiroshi's fractured compass, its needle eternally quivering at 192° - the precise angle the old forester had snapped it during their last argument over "measurable mysticism." Sarah's mandala developed a stress fracture when morning dew dissolved hidden ink from her trouser pocket notebook, revealing tomorrow's schedule now bleeding into fern rhizomes.

"Beautiful disruption," Kenji observed, his chrysanthemum tea steam warping air currents to send a maple seed helicoptering into Sarah's hair. She froze mid-correction, fingers inches from enforcing order, when the pine chose that moment to drop a resin globule onto her Burberry belt's silver buckle. The viscous splash spread slowly, consuming her corporate insignia under amber hegemony.

By third rotation, Sarah's mandala breathed like

a living balance sheet gone feral. Japanese maple leaves overlapped in hostile takeover patterns. Acorn caps hosted miniature moss rebellions. When Lachlan placed the final asymmetrical touch - a snapped twig angled at 73° - Sarah's exhale carried the weight of thirty-seven quarterly reports.

"More interesting," she admitted, the admission fracturing something behind her sternum. Kenji's mugwort infusion steamed approval across the mandala's northeast quadrant. Hana's charcoal stick drifted into the circle, adding shadow where light demanded dominance. And Aisha, silent until now, pressed a cracked sidewalk fragment from her ginkgo's domain into the composition's flawed heart.

The forest approved through shifted light - sunbeams now highlighting imperfections like coveted artisanal flaws in corporate pottery. Sarah's abandoned belt became a compass rose pointing only to true north of chaos, while Hiroshi's broken instrument hummed approval against Lachlan's flask. Somewhere beyond the clearing, a woodpecker began auditing pine bark accounts with deliberate, irregular rhythm.

The elm's bark bronchioles pressed against

Kenji's palms, each ridge conducting arboreal respirations that mocked his spirometer charts. His grandfather's herb pouch swung metronome-like, dried mitsuba leaves ticking off the seconds since his last preventative inhaler puff.

"Speak to the apothecary," Lachlan urged, pressing Kenji's left thumb into a sap well warm as childhood fevers. The elm's roots still cradled shards of Edo-era medicine bottles, their cobalt glass patterns replicated in the dappled shadows climbing Kenji's arms.

"I monitor sleep cycles. Track pollen counts. Calculate..." His clinical cadence faltered as cicada nymphs stirred beneath their feet, seventeen-year hibernation schedules vibrating through shoe soles. The elm responded with a resin droplet that hit his collar - 98.6°F, same as his mother's worried palm during asthma attacks.

Lachlan guided Kenji's hands into the root mudra - pinkies earthbound, thumbs arcing like exhaling lungs. The position stretched scar tissue from IV ports in a way that unearthed suppressed memories: cherry blossom forecasts scrolling on hospital TVs while machines beeped his survival probabilities.

As Kenji confessed medication side effects, the elm unleashed a pollen plume that danced around his inhaler's propellant cloud in a waltz of competing remedies. Mugwort from his grandfather's pouch began absorbing palm sweat, activating phytochemicals that darkened in real-time like mood ring betrayal.

"Would you begrudge a sapling its crooked growth?" Lachlan's question coincided with a cicada's emergence hole collapsing under Kenji's knee. The elm's leaves filtered sunlight into clinical fluorescence, then softened to grandmother's shamisen evening lullabies as mycoglobin threads began binding his stress hormones into new fungal architectures.

When Kenji's breathing finally synced with the elm's sap rise, the tree commemorated the moment with an acorn dropped precisely onto his pharmaceutical spreadsheets. The impact scattered numbers into configurations resembling his grandfather's handwritten herb lore - equations no peer review panel could parse, but that his alveoli understood completely.

The willow's branches wrote anarchic haiku across Hana's sketchbook, inky tendrils overwriting years of precisely measured negative space. Lachlan knelt at the tree's base, burning fistfuls of gallery rejection letters whose ashes spiraled upward to form kanji even the wind couldn't translate.

"Movement bypasses the critic's knife," he declared, pressing a smoldering twig to Hana's charcoal stick. The tip flared crimson - temporary liberation from graphite's monochrome prison.

Her first gestures came stiff as marionette limbs, elbow angles mirroring the RISD life drawing instructor who'd slapped a ruler across her wrist for "excessive contour deviation." The willow retaliated by catching her sleeve mid-stroke, unraveling yarn strands into something resembling Hiroshi's bamboo flute ties.

When afternoon gusts tore her hair bun loose, the liberated strands danced like grandmother's silver-streaked tresses during Obon festivals. Hana's feet moved unbidden, crushing abandoned charcoal into moss cushions that released spores in standing ovation puffs. A phalanx of carpenter ants ascended her ankle, their antennae translating her calf muscles' tremors into a pheromone review: *More spirals. Less rulers.*

Lachlan's flask lay angled to reflect her teenage graffiti masterpiece - a Shinjuku underpass mural later whitewashed by city workers. In the warped silver, Hana saw her hands transform into the willow's green-sapped brushes, painting light across stone in strokes that would give her former gallerist hives.

By the time cicadas began vespers, her motions had dissolved into pure dendrologic response. The willow's branches applauded in papery whispers, scattering catkins that adhered to her sweat-damp neck like botanical medals of honor. Somewhere beyond the grove, a Tokyo art collector's chihuahua sneezed at the seismic shift in avant-garde weather patterns.

The ginkgo's roots cradled Aisha's corporate heels in cracked concrete palms, its fan-shaped leaves translating subway vibrations into Kampala thunderstorm rhythms. She unrolled barkcloth paper imprinted with grandmother's fingerprints, the mwanyi tree fibers still humming with songs from the Naguru papermaking hut.

Her fountain pen stalled - Ugandan robusta

coffee ink refusing to mingle with cedar resin additive. When a cicada husk fell as misplaced punctuation, Aisha heard her uncle's voice reading ministerial decrees that banned moonlight gatherings. The ginkgo answered by pushing its roots against her soles, conducting memories of colonial survey maps dissolving under mau-mau urine.

"Write the lies first," Lachlan advised, pressing his flask cap into service as a soil scoop. The stainless steel remembered Hiroshi's thumbprints and twelve failed research proposals.

Aisha's first words bled into the paper's thirsty fibers: *Forgive me for shrinking*. The ginkgo pulsed in approval, its roots cracking a new sidewalk segment that mirrored her childhood scar from falling through a British irrigation grate. When tears diluted the ink into Africa's coastline, carpenter ants shouldered the brine-laden droplets to their queen as ceremonial offering.

She buried the confession where feeder roots throbbed with tomorrow's growth, Lachlan's flask cap leaving corporate logo indentations in the humus. The group's hands descended - Sarah's pine-resined fingers, Kenji's herb-stained palms, Hana's charcoal-calloused tips - their combined warmth jumpstarting mycorrhizal encryption protocols older than colonial languages.

As twilight shifted tectonic plates, the ginkgo's chlorophyll began translating Aisha's sorrow into xylem sonnets. Somewhere in Nakawa, a surviving mwanyi tree dropped a seedpod onto a developer's Mercedes hood.

Lachlan's cedar wore his academic failures as ceremonial scars, sap-sealed equations from abandoned theses glowing amber under the forest's forensic gaze. He pressed his spine against the trunk where Hiroshi's chisel had once gouged *Unscientific!* in Meiji-era kanji, now subsumed by decades of compensatory growth rings.

"They called it 'folkloric methodology'," he confessed, snapping a charcoal pencil that remembered thirty-seven grant rejection margins. Fire ants mobilized to cart away the graphite shards, rearranging them into myrmecophytic critiques of peer review culture.

His whiskey flask sweated droplets containing

molecular ghosts - melted nameplates from conferences where colleagues praised his "quaint animist charm" between cocktails. The cedar responded by oozing resin around a nest of paper wasps building cells from his shredded tenure application.

When Lachlan imitated his doctoral advisor's nasal dismissal of "tree whispering pseudoscience," a nuthatch hammered Morse-code approval against the trunk. The vibration dislodged a moth whose wing patterns diagrammed the exact neural pathway where impostor syndrome metastasizes.

By the time he described sabotaging his own spectrometer to preserve a cedar's dignity, Hana's charcoal had transcribed his words into bark-script marginalia. Sarah's pine needle tears and Kenji's antihistamine spray formed salt-crystal lenses magnifying Hiroshi's final journal entry - *True science embraces what instruments cannot grasp.*

The forest documented his confession in cross-species collaboration: squirrels cached acorns in syllabic clusters, orb weavers strung validation traps, and the cedar's roots transmitted pulse-coded absolution to every mycorrhizal terminal in the grove.

Twilight distilled the group's transformations into a forest apothecary - Sarah's pine needle tincture bubbling with liberated office hours, Kenji's elm pods rattling ancestral prescriptions, Hana's willow charcoal rods pregnant with unsanctioned light.

Lachlan poured cedar-infused whisky into Hiroshi's bamboo timepiece, the liquor flowing through 108 hand-carved notches that now measured growth rings instead of minutes. Sarah's Burberry belt coiled around a nurse log, its buckle oxidizing into a sundial gnomon that tracked time through canopy apertures rather than Outlook alerts.

As Kenji buried expired antihistamines beneath his elm's pharmacopeia skirt, cicada nymphs began converting the plastic vials into vibrational amplifiers for their 2038 emergence symphony. Aisha's silk scarf dissolved into mycelial lattices, the jasmine threads now conducting Kampala's red soil electricity to the ginkgo's concrete battlefront.

Hana's sketchbook lay open to a willow-dictated manifesto, its pages fluttering in breeze patterns that erased former gallery coordinates. When fireflies congregated to illuminate her marginalia, their abdomens flashed in precise critique of Shibuya's light pollution statutes.

Lachlan's final cedar sprig joined the bundle, its resin sealing their pact in chemical Braille. The forest celebrated through cross-species collaboration - woodpeckers drumming tenure revocation notices into snag flesh, slugs trailblazing over dissolved corporate letterhead, and the mycorrhizal network compiling their stories into humus folios.

As the first stars pierced the canopy, Hiroshi's bamboo chimes stirred from dormancy, their tones mapping the invisible architecture connecting Sarah's mandala imperfections to Kampala's mango root rebellions. The taniwha flask grinned its tarnished approval, already filling with next season's revelations.

The Confluence of Science and Spirit

Dawn's fingers pried apart cedar boughs with surgical precision, spotlighting the stump lectern where Lachlan McGregor pinned cortisol graphs using cicada exuviae. The forest had dressed for trial - sugar maple leaves curled like plaintiff exhibits, their scarlet veins mirroring the rise-fall-rise of Sarah's stress markers plotted nearby. He adjusted a shard of mica beneath the "After" column, its schist layers catching light at angles that made the nosediving data points spark like fireworks dying mid-descent.

Three Japanese maple saplings bowed under the weight of his evidence - immune cell counts transcribed on birch bark scrolls, their edges charred from hasty campfire revisions. A spotted salamander served as paperweight for Hana's before-and-after sketches, its amphibious belly leaving damp ellipses where gallery rejection letters once dominated.

Lachlan's whiskey flask sweated approval into a hollow scooped by woodpecker persistence, its taniwha engraving fogged with phytoncide-rich condensation.

"Bleeding heart," he murmured, thumbing a trillium's petals into position beside Kenji's allergy meds spreadsheet. The flower's crimson drips mirrored the plummeting red spikes of histamine levels. Somewhere overhead, a nuthatch began hammering its endorsement into shagbark hickory.

Dr. Blackwood's approach registered first in the soil - Vibram soles compressing moss colonies evolved to withstand samurai marches. She emerged through trembling ferns clutching a notebook whose pages fluttered like surrendered white flags, its binding threads blooming with embroidery fungi. Gone were the tablet's predatory angles; this was paper that remembered being trees.

"You've...redecorated," she observed, Montblanc hovering over cortisol curves. A ladybug traversed the "Before" column's peak, wings folding salute to its conquered elevation.

Lachlan nudged a galls inkwell toward her. "The data grows more honest when rooted." His smile deepened as she sniffed the oak apple infusion - half challenge, half invitation.

The forest deployed its welcoming committee. Sarah arrived with hickory nuts spilling from blazer pockets, lapels adorned with white pine resin medals that outshone her former corporate pins. Kenji's arrival sneeze scattered goldenrod pollen across his medical charts in abstract affirmation. When Hana pressed a charcoal-rubbed fist to Blackwood's notebook, the resulting thumbprint contained entire growth rings of unspoken apologies.

Aisha completed the circle by depositing a fractured parking meter head at the stump's base, its rusty entrails spilling onto immune response timelines. "Urban mycorrhizal network," she declared, Kampala vowels softening the steel carcass' edges.

Blackwood's pen hesitated—then dove, documenting the scene in margins wide enough for miracles. Above them, the cedar's branches shifted sunspot spotlights, conducting a defense no peer review panel could impeach.

Lachlan unscrewed the firefly jar with a winemaker's reverence, releasing bioluminescent jurors to inspect the data. Their abdomen flares pulsed in time with Sarah's vanished midnight cortisol spikes—three quick flashes for every vanished anxiety attack. He tracked one particularly ardent defender circling the NK cell proliferation chart, its cold light burnishing the 73% increase into something resembling celestial cartography.

"The numbers sing better outdoors," he admitted, sweeping an alder branch pointer across laminated sheets. Evening primrose petals marked key inflection points—their solar-yellow faces tilted toward Blackwood's furrowed brow. "Peer-reviewed journals prefer sterile columns, but the stream prefers..."

He nudged a pebble into the water. Ripples rearranged themselves into logarithmic curves mirroring Kenji's immunoglobulin surge. A water strider adjusted its stance, middle legs indicating p-values with arachnid precision.

"Circadian heresy," Blackwood muttered, though her pen's frantic scratching betrayed fascination. When a firefly settled on her "Marginal Error" notation, she didn't brush it off but added an asterisk: *Lampyridae corroboration.*

Sarah's contribution emerged via cracked smartphone, its screen casting lunar schematics across gathered faces. "Fourteen months ago," she began, thumbing to a graph where crimson peaks mimicked earthquake seismographs. "Board meeting Mondays versus..." The swipe revealed a placid lake of blues—sleep architecture rebuilt by white pine lullabies. A caterpillar inched approval across the charging port.

Kenji's evidence unfolded like a medicinal scroll. "Seventy-three inhaler puffs last autumn," he recited, pressed gentian florets marking each rescue dose. Beside them lay this season's tally—seven violet petals floating in the ghostly wake of mugwort tea stewardship. His grandfather's spectacles fogged at the differential.

The forest interjected its testimony. A pileated woodpecker drummed rapid-fire peer review on black locust heartwood, each staccato burst challenging methodology. Lachlan answered by unleashing a sugar maple spinner—"Wind direction during cortisol sampling"—its descent arc silencing avian critique.

When Blackwood's pen rolled into fresh fox tracks, she left it nestled beside fern fiddleheads. "Your control group..."

"...Wears asphalt shoes and fluorescent

162

lighting," Aisha interjected, spreading rooftop garden photos where broccoli florets erupted through chainlink restraint. "The control is coming."

As dusk blurred data into intuition, the fireflies convened their verdict in blinking semaphore. Lachlan's flask made rounds, whiskey now fermented with answers no IRB could censure. Somewhere downstream, the water strider began calculating their next breakthrough.

The cedar wore its history in braille - shrapnel scars from Shōwa-era bombardments, sap-sealed bullet holes that sang in minor keys when winds blew from the sea. Lachlan pressed Blackwood's palm against a furrow where postwar saplings had swallowed ration cans whole, her lifeline intersecting dendrochronology's ledger of resilience.

"Forehead here," he guided, positioning her where morning sun had baked centuries of priestly petitions into the bark. Her Valentino blouse caught on burls shaped like fetal dragons. "Breathe like you're apologizing to someone."

The forest leaned closer. Sarah counted aloud

in the forgotten cadence of lullabies while Kenji's sneezes marked time in pollen-rich intervals. Blackwood's first exhalation misted the tree's fissures - a humid offering that stirred ambrosia beetles from their hexagonal chambers. By breath twelve, her Rolex fogged into uselessness. At thirty-three, a cambium tremor traveled her spine's corporate curvature.

Hana documented the metamorphosis in lichen pigments - ultramarine for tension's ebb, iron oxide for emerging wonder. When Blackwood's knees buckled at seventy-four, the cedar compensated by oozing analgesic resins where her shins met earth.

The forest tallied the remainder in winged arithmetic - eight chickadee warning calls, three falling ginkgo blades, seventeen cicada thrum intervals. As the 108th breath escaped, a wood ant deposited a fir needle crown at Blackwood's Louboutin, its resin still warm from the tree's approval.

"I... There was..." Blackwood's fingers worried a tenure application's edge in her satchel before releasing it to the dirt. The document absorbed cedar dew as Hana unveiled canvases where living moss spelled "SOLD" in Myxomycete script.

Aisha's smartphone resurrection showcased dandelion guerrillas breaching parking garage ramparts. "Your concrete control group," she smiled, playbutton activating a video where chickweed devoured chainlink fencing at stop-motion pace.

Lachlan uncapped his flask over Blackwood's discarded pen, whiskey blending with cedar tears to seal their collaboration. Somewhere beyond the clearing, Hiroshi's ghost laughed through bamboo chimes as the first owl feather landed on their data, its barred patterning echoing both dendrograms and surrender.

The Forest's Embrace

Twilight pressed its thumb against the cedar canopy, squeezing last light through needle-filtered apertures. Lachlan's boot scuffed a crescent in the duff, his nostrils flaring at the pine's anticipatory resin burst - sharp as Sarah's abandoned perfume but warmer, alive with terpene promises. Somewhere beyond the nurse log altar, a veery's evening aria dissolved into the space between heartbeats where rituals began.

Sarah arrived first, her Burberry trench hanging open to reveal blouse sleeves rolled above wrists still imprinted with spreadsheet-grid tan lines. The pine awaited her like a prickly suitor, its bark plates arranged in fractals that mocked corporate organizational charts. She pressed a palm to the vertical crack splitting its western face - a lightning scar from the same August storm that had flooded her Tribeca office basement, destroying six months of market analytics. The tree breathed cinnamon defense chemicals against her cuticles.

Kenji materialized through fern shadows, grandfather's herb pouch clinking against pharmaceutical inhalers. His elm presided over a rebel apothecary - mugwort colonizing asphalt seams, dandelions hoarding cortisone in fuzzy seed heads. The trunk's smooth southern face still bore charcoal equations from a Meiji-era cough syrup trials. His sneeze scattered goldenrod pollen across the ritual circle, each grain adhering to his collar's starch lines like nature's bullet points.

Hana's willow trailed sorrow in catkin tassels, branches dipping to caress her charcoal-stained knuckles. She tilted her head at the precise angle captured in her infamous "Urban Arboricides" installation - the same pose that had earned the Mori Museum's reprimand for "excessive anthropomorphism." A breeze rearranged the canopy's green hair to match her abandoned sketch of Tokyo's suffocated saplings, graphite smears dissolving into living patterns.

Aisha's ginkgo rose defiant from concrete carnage, roots swelling beneath imported sidewalk slabs. Her Prada mule nudged a fractured paver, revealing mycelial lacework digesting polymer binders. The leaves fanned golden approval, their fan shapes mirroring grandmother's medicinal herb charts drawn in red Uganda clay. When her phone buzzed final condo board rejection notices, the sapling dropped a seedpod on the screen, embryonic roots already probing glass cracks.

"Watch your step, the phoebes nested late this year," Lachlan cautioned, brushing owl feathers into compass points. His whiskey flask sweated ancestral promises onto the offering stone - twelve generations of McGregor botanists whispering through peat smoke. As he unrolled Hiroshi's bamboo breath counter, the notches caught firefly light glowing green as Sarah's abandoned spreadsheet cells.

"Right palms over heartwood scars," he instructed, pressing his own hand to black locust bark striated like Hana's charcoal strokes. The group shuffled into alignment, Aisha's bare toes curling around ginkgo roots while Kenji's oxfords crushed valerian into numbing salve. When the first star pierced the canopy, Lachlan's whisper carried the weight of thirty-seven failed rituals: "Breathe like you're apologizing to someone still listening."

Above them, the willow sighed in maternal A-flat, its branches lowering to catch Hana's falling hairpin. Somewhere beyond the clearing, concrete continued its slow surrender.

Bark pores dilated beneath Sarah's forehead, drinking salt and foundation as the pine's cambium layer pulsed like a carotid artery. Somewhere beyond her spreadsheet-tuned eardrum, Lachlan's voice threaded through xylem channels: "Your anger makes interesting fertilizer." Her left stiletto sank deeper into loam, sole bonding with mycorrhizal subpoenas.

Kenji's elbows locked mid-mudra, grandfather's spectacles sliding down a nose greasy with antihistamine sweat. The elm's northern face bore a concave depression from decades of herbalists pressing foreheads to its pharmacy trunk. His inhaler canister rolled against mugwort clusters, its albuterol mist mingling with elecampane's bronchial promises. Breath hitched at thirty-seven - the exact number of rejected asthma studies in his CV - until bark flavonoids dilated airways better than any peer-reviewed molecule.

Hana's fingers spidered across willow ribs, charcoal smudges aligning with lenticels exhaling oxygenic sonnets. The tree mirrored her tremor-forge grip, catkins brushing pulse points in time with Lachlan's count. "Your lines flow better when wet," he observed, sprinkling whisky across her paper. Pigment bled into cambium, tattooing the willow with shadows of her condemned Shibuya mural.

"Fifth cycle - expand those corporate lungs," Lachlan prompted, taniwha flask trailing peat smoke across Aisha's roots. Her bare soles curled around ginkgo rhytidome, urban callouses meeting dendriform ridges that mapped Kampala's red dirt roads. Concrete particulates fell like confetti as the sapling's vascular hum synchronized with grandmother's banana leaf fan stirring monsoon air.

Sarah's blouse seam split with a sigh, releasing thirty-eight months of boardroom posture into photosynthetic embrace. The pine injected her deltoids with relaxed lignins, amber droplets crystallizing along spine meridians where stress once pooled. When her watch alarm chirped a stock market reminder, wood ants disassembled the circuitry with pincer precision.

By breath seventy-two, the forest conducted their exhalations. Kenji's wheeze transformed into elm's transpiration gust, Hana's charcoal sighs darkening willow's twilight tears. Firefly abdomens flashed green approval - three pulses for Aisha's root network expansion, seven for Sarah's abandoned Outlook passwords dissolving into humus.

"Ninety-one... ninety-two..." Lachlan's count dissolved into mycelial mathematics as owl feathers marked completed cycles. Somewhere beneath them, the cedar's taproot transmitted approval through shared groundwater - Hiroshi's laughter echoing through aquifer caverns where data streams surrendered to xylem truth.

Sarah's heartbeat thrummed through pine rings, each contraction pumping resin through corporate veinwork. When she gasped, the tree answered with a sugar surge that caramelized seven years of stored tension audits. Somewhere in her abandoned briefcase, termites began translating stock reports into nursery rhymes.

Kenji's elbows unlocked as elm larixinol derivatives metabolized his pharmaceutical load. The tree's sap pulse sang through his radial artery - ancient decongestant lullabies outprescribing Merck manuals. His final antihistamine capsule dissolved against tongue papillae, replaced by mugwort's bitter truth.

The willow branch tapped Hana's temple in 3/4 time, conducting charcoal memories through catkin batons. Her sketch hand moved unbidden, capturing the exact moment corporate commissions decomposed into mycorrhizal marginalia. When tears diluted india ink into sepia tones, the willow's roots absorbed salt testimony through osmotic forgiveness.

Aisha's ginkgo transmitted subway vibrations up through metatarsals, each tremor a telegram from Tokyo's buried rivers. The tree's fan leaves applauded her Kampala vowels reshaping themselves around Japanese phonemes - linguistic mycelia bridging continents through shared chloroplast.

At breath 108, the forest inhaled their collective surrender. Pine needles fell like stock tickers. Elm pollen dusted pharmaceutical patents. Willow catkins erased gallery contracts. Ginkgo seeds cracked concrete's monopoly.

Lachlan's whiskey flask caught their exhalations in amber suspension - Sarah's quarterly panic, Kenji's bronchial fear, Hana's rejected authenticity, Aisha's transplanted roots. The taniwha engraving pulsed approval, its jade eyes reflecting not what they'd lost, but what the trees had always known they'd find.

Carrying the Forest Home

Morning arrived through the cedar canopy in coins of light, each photon aged seven minutes from solar surface to forest floor, where Lachlan arranged objects on a moss-furred stone with the care of a museum curator handling prayer beads. His weathered hands placed bamboo boxes beside coils of twine, pressed flower papers, and glass vials that caught the light like captured phytoncides, while around him the ancient grove exhaled its approval in resinous whispers. A crow's shadow flickered across his work surface, its wings beating time with the pulse still thrumming in his temples from last night's ritual—108 breaths that had dissolved more than atmospheric carbon.

Sarah approached first, her gait no longer the metronomic clip of quarterly reports but something softer, heel-to-toe rolling like the river stones she'd learned to read. The Burberry hung open, its belt abandoned somewhere between breaths seventy and seventy-one, revealing a blouse whose sleeves bore pine resin stains like medals of a different kind of service. She crouched beside the display, fingers hovering over objects with the hesitation of someone relearning how to choose without spreadsheets.

"The stone chooses you as much as you choose it," Lachlan murmured, watching her palm settle over a river-smoothed oval of granite, its surface holding the exact temperature of decision. The stone's weight pressed into her lifeline—forty-three grams of geological patience worn smooth by ten thousand years of current. Pine needles from her tree ally clung to her sleeve cuff, and she gathered them with movements that would have seemed foreign to the woman who'd arrived clutching tablets and calculators.

"This stone has trusted you, Sarah." Lachlan's eyes crinkled at corners mapped by decades of squinting through forest light. "Keep it close during those board meetings. Let them wonder why you're smiling at quarterly projections."

She turned the stone over, thumb finding a depression that matched her grip perfectly, as if erosion had anticipated this moment. The pine needles she selected weren't the greenest or straightest but the ones bearing tiny punctures from boring beetles—imperfect, resilient, honest about their survival.

Kenji's approach announced itself through the absence of wheeze, his breathing clear as the morning air that carried hints of wild mint from the understory. Grandfather's herb pouch swung against his hip, but the pharmaceutical inhaler remained buried beneath handkerchiefs he no longer needed. His fingers moved with inherited precision, selecting elm bark strips whose inner cambium still wept medicinal sap.

"That one's from the lightning scar," Lachlan noted as Kenji peeled a section bearing charred edges. "Your grandfather would have called it twice-blessed—once by the tree's growth, once by heaven's touch."

The younger man's laugh carried no bitter aftertaste of bronchodilators. He gathered mugwort leaves with the reverence of someone who'd learned to breathe through green filters rather than plastic ones, adding lamb's quarters and plantain to his collection. Each plant specimen went into rice paper envelopes he'd folded himself, corners precise as origami cranes but somehow more alive.

176

Hana materialized from behind the willow curtain, charcoal dust beneath her fingernails transformed from mark of shame to badge of honor. Her selections came swift and certain— willow twigs that curved like question marks, maple leaves whose yellows bled into oranges with the recklessness of watercolor accidents. She no longer arranged them in rigid patterns but let them fall into her collecting cloth as they wished, chaos becoming its own composition.

"Your lines flow like sap now," Lachlan observed, producing his leather journal to demonstrate leaf-pressing technique. The maple leaf he chose bore insect damage that transformed its surface into lace, pressing it between pages already thick with forest memories. "See how the holes become part of the design? Gallery walls never understood that kind of honesty."

Aisha's bare feet had found every root and stone between the ginkgo grove and here, her designer shoes dangling from one hand like shed skins. She selected her ginkgo leaf with the focus of someone choosing ammunition for a revolution—golden, fan-shaped, with enough substance to survive being pressed between permit applications and zoning maps. The moss sample she scraped from concrete chunks spoke of victories measured in millimeters, of life refusing to honor property lines.

"Urban moss carries different songs," Lachlan said, helping her wrap the sample in damp cotton. "It knows about carbon monoxide and dog piss but also about rain channeling off glass towers, about the persistence of spores in hostile territory."

The photography ritual unfolded in reverent silence. Sarah's phone, cracked screen refracting pine bark into prismatic honesty. Kenji's grandfather's box camera clicking mechanical approval of elm portraits. Hana's quick sketches serving as viewfinder for moments no lens could capture. Aisha's architectural eye framing ginkgo against skyline ghosts.

When Lachlan produced the flask, its contents had darkened to the amber of fossilized resin, cedar essence marrying whiskey in ways that would horrify purists and delight trees. The metal caught morning light, taniwha scales seeming to swim through new liquid territories.

"To finding the forest," he began, voice roughened by either emotion or cedar tannins, "even when we're far from trees. To board meetings interrupted by pine memories. To galleries that smell of willow. To medicine found in grandmother's footsteps. To cities that crack their concrete smiles."

The flask passed hand to hand, each sip a communion with place and time and the peculiar magic of humans remembering they were never separate from the breathing world. Above them, the cedars leaned in to witness this closing ceremony, their crowns filtering light into benedictions that would follow each person home, pressed between pages, caught in glass, carried in pockets where phones once ruled.

When the circle broke, it reformed in wider rings—Sarah's stone warm against her palm, Kenji's herbs rustling promises, Hana's twigs scripting new alphabets, Aisha's moss dreaming of vertical gardens. The forest had given them its vocabulary. Now they would return to cities and spreadsheets and galleries and bureaucracies, carrying seeds of a different kind of literacy.

Sarah's office on the forty-third floor had never known soil, its surfaces evolved for the sterile efficiency of quarterly reports and merger documents, which made the appearance of potting mix beneath her manicured nails feel like small-scale insurrection as she nestled a hart's-tongue fern between the Keurig machine and her corporate excellence awards. The cleaning staff had given up questioning the transformation—first the pine branch in a crystal vase, then the river stone paperweight that left mineral rings on acquisition contracts, now this botanical invasion that turned her workspace into something between boardroom and greenhouse.

She adjusted a philodendron's angle to catch the afternoon light, its heart-shaped leaves trembling with the building's HVAC exhale. From her laptop, a soundscape of Japanese forest rain competed with the distant ring of market bells, the audio file labeled simply "Tuesday 3PM Sanity.mp3" in her meticulously organized folders. The plant's aerial roots reached toward her desk lamp like a child seeking warmth, and she found herself pausing mid-email to watch their almost imperceptible growth.

"I swear this philodendron hears my deadlines," she murmured to the empty office, fingers brushing a leaf that released the faintest scent of earth into the recycled air. The stone

180

from Kyoto sat beside her keyboard, its weight anchoring something primal while pie charts bloomed across her screen in colors that suddenly seemed garish compared to the subtle green variations in her botanical audience.

Her assistant knocked, paused at the threshold. "The Singapore team is ready for the—is that moss?"

"Mood moss," Sarah confirmed, misting a shallow dish where emerald cushions transformed a discarded lucite award base into something approaching art. "It changes color with humidity. More reliable than market indicators."

The forest sounds swelled—a woodpecker's percussion underlying her typing rhythm, her breathing unconsciously syncing with the recorded wind through cedars. When her phone buzzed with urgent notifications, she let it ring, watching instead how the philodendron's newest leaf uncurled with patient determination, each day revealing another centimeter of green truth in the fluorescent wilderness.

Dawn in Riverside Park found Kenji's breath clouding around a hand-drawn map, his fingers steady despite the October chill as he pinned laminated herb specimens to predetermined points along gravel paths. The mugwort sample went near the memorial bench where arthritis sufferers gathered, plantain stationed by the playground where knees got scraped, wild mint marking the overlook where his elderly neighbor, Mrs. Chen, practiced tai chi with lungs that rattled like maracas.

"You're early today, Doctor," she wheezed, though he'd told her a dozen times he wasn't that kind of doctor, just someone who'd learned to listen to plants the way his grandfather had listened to symptoms.

"Taste this," he said, crushing spearmint between his fingers, the oils releasing sharp enough to cut through her cigarette-scarred airways. The plant grew wild near the pond, thriving on goose droppings and joggers' lost ambitions. "Just the leaves, not the stem. Steep for three minutes, no more."

Her skeptical sniff transformed as the menthol compounds hit her sinuses. "Smells like my mother's cough remedy, but..." She gestured at the dewy leaves. "This grows here? In the city?"

"Especially in the city," Kenji confirmed, his grandfather's watch ticking approval against his wrist. "Plants adapt. They learn concrete the way they once learned volcanic soil. This mint? It's filtering bus exhaust, transforming poison into medicine."

By the time full daylight arrived, a small crowd had gathered—dog walkers and pre-work joggers drawn by the spectacle of someone mapping healing in a landscape they'd relegated to backdrop. Kenji's newest inhaler remained buried in his jacket, untouched for seven weeks now, while his hands distributed photocopied guides decorated with pressed specimens and his grandmother's marginal notes translated into English.

"The elm by the boat house has shelf mushrooms," he pointed northeast, where the tree's pharmacy spread itself in fungal shelves. "Not for eating, but seeing them means the tree's recycling its own medicine. Like a forest emergency room, always open."

Mrs. Chen's laugh came clearer already, mint molecules opening passages that privilege and prescriptions had failed to reach.

Hana's studio in Queens still smelled of turpentine and failure, but now cedar shavings sweetened the mix, scattered across tables where stretched canvases had once awaited the violent precision of her urban landscapes. The charcoal-smudged apron, veteran of a thousand frustrated sessions, now bore the brown-black streaks of soil and oak gall ink, its pockets bulging with twigs that clattered like fortune-telling bones when she moved.

Natural light fell across her work table—she'd removed the blackout curtains that had protected her pieces from UV damage, inviting the sun to participate in whatever emerged from bark and paper. A frame meant for her cancelled gallery show now housed a collection of pressed maple leaves, their insect damage transformed into a study on negative space that would have made her professors weep with either joy or horror.

"Structure is overrated," she told the willow branch she'd been sketching for three hours, its curves defying every composition rule beaten into her at art school. The drawing emerged not through controlled strokes but through a conversation between charcoal and chance—here a knot became an eye, there a split in the bark suggested the arch of a spine in repose.

Her phone, buried under sketches of sidewalk weeds, buzzed with a reminder about the Guggenheim submission deadline. Instead of diving for it, she pressed a fresh sheet of handmade paper against the window where city rain had left mineral deposits. The resulting print would never hang in climate-controlled galleries, but it contained something her previous work had lacked—the honest collaboration between human intention and materials that carried their own memories.

When her landlord knocked about the smell, she opened the door wearing twigs in her hair like a crown, explaining how the fermentation process of making oak gall ink connected her to medieval illuminators. He retreated, muttering about artists, while behind her the studio transformed into something between laboratory and forest floor, where failure became compost for whatever wanted to grow.

The sidewalk outside the Harlem subway stop bore the usual signatures of urban defeat—gum melanomas, urine stains, the geometric scars of replaced concrete squares that never quite matched their neighbors. Aisha crouched where the bodega's runoff created a microclimate, her mud-flecked sketchpad balanced on one knee while she drew another pocket forest into being, pencil lines transforming blank walls into vertical gardens that existed, for now, only in graphite and determination.

Her Prada mules, the ones that had traversed Kyoto's moss, now bore the honorable scars of community board meetings and contractor site visits. The permit application numbers she jotted in margins read like poetry to those who understood their power—LPC-2847B (historic district variance), NYC-DOT-3921 (sidewalk modification), CERT-ENV-8832 (environmental impact waiver). Each number a small victory in the bureaucratic aikido required to bring green to concrete.

"Whatchu drawing, miss?" A teenager paused, basketball tucked under one arm, drawn perhaps by the incongruity of someone in designer clothes kneeling on Lenox Avenue with dirt under her nails.

"Your future," Aisha replied, tilting the sketchpad to reveal climbing vines conquering a brick wall, planters spilling from fire escapes, moss writing its own graffiti across abandoned lots. "See that corner? Imagine ginkgo trees. Those windows? Picture morning glories climbing up, purple flowers you could see from the train."

The kid squinted, and for a moment she saw it reflected in his eyes—the neighborhood not as it was but as it could be, when concrete learned to breathe and walls became vertical forests. He nodded once, solemn as a convert, before bouncing his ball away into the urban percussion that Aisha now heard differently, each impact a possibility for roots to find new cracks.

Her phone mapped fifty-seven potential sites between here and the river, each annotated with soil samples she'd smuggled in perfume bottles, pH tested in her kitchen sink. The forest had taught her patience measured in growth rings. The city would learn it too, one permit at a time.

Dusk arrived at the teahouse like a careful guest, removing its shoes of harsh daylight at the threshold where inside and outside dissolved into paper screens and shadow puppets, while Lachlan arranged writing materials on the low table with movements learned from Hiroshi—patient, deliberate, trusting that ceremony could hold what words alone could not. The garden beyond whispered through its repertoire of evening sounds: water trickling across stones worn smooth by twenty generations of contemplation, bamboo fountain filling and tipping in mechanical meditation, crickets tuning their instruments for nocturnal symphony.

The others entered as they had learned to enter forests—Sarah's corporate armor left with her shoes, Kenji's breathing already synchronized with the fountain's rhythm, Hana's fingers traced the wall's wood grain like reading braille scriptures, Aisha's bare feet finding the warm spots where afternoon sun still lived in tatami mat fiber. They arranged themselves around the table where Lachlan had placed sheets of handmade paper, each piece containing visible plant fibers like captured veins, alongside brushes worn smooth by generations of letter writers and small clay pots of ink that smelled of rain and char.

"Write to your future self," Lachlan instructed, his voice carrying the same tone he'd used teaching them to read bark—serious but not solemn, sacred but not severe. "Not just promises, but reminders of how the forest made you feel. How your bones learned to breathe. How spreadsheets became leaf patterns. How gallery walls dissolved into willow shadows."

He demonstrated with his own brush, the ink flowing like sap as he drew characters that meant both "remember" and "return." The

188

sound of brush on paper became the room's heartbeat—soft scratches and whispers as thoughts transformed into marks that would outlive the moment.

Sarah's brush hesitated before making contact, a bead of ink trembling at its tip like morning dew deciding whether to fall. When she finally wrote, the characters came firm and clear: "Strength lives in stillness." She elaborated in margins that spiraled like fern fronds, describing board meetings where she would hold her river stone beneath the table, its coolness reminding her that quarterly projections were just another kind of weather, passing through. Her letter spoke of learning to read the exhaustion in colleagues' shoulders the way she'd learned to read drought stress in pine needles, of replacing coffee breaks with window-gazing meditations where pigeons became as significant as profit margins.

Kenji's pharmacist hands moved with prescription precision, but the words that emerged spoke of medicine beyond capsules. He wrote of dawn walks where he would teach neighbors to taste the morning air for allergen warnings, to find plantain for bee stings in sidewalk cracks. His letter contained sketches of the medicinal garden he would plant at the

189

community center, each herb labeled with both Latin names and his grandmother's nicknames. "The real healing," he wrote in a margin, "happens when people stop being afraid of their own breathing."

Hana's charcoal-trained fingers gripped the brush like a weapon surrendering its violence. Her letters came out part text, part drawing—words dissolving into images of gallery walls breached by living vines. She documented her plan to leave frames empty for shadows to complete, to invite viewers to contribute their own found objects to installations. "The forest taught me that control is just another word for fear," she wrote, the ink bleeding slightly where her tear had fallen, the imperfection making the words more true.

Aisha's letter unfolded like architectural blueprints translated into poetry. She wrote of permits as prayers, of bureaucracy as another kind of forest to navigate with patience and cunning. Her words mapped a city where every empty lot could host a pocket wilderness, where fire escapes dripped with tomato vines and morning glories. She included sketches of modular planters that could transform overnight, guerrilla gardens that would appear like mushrooms after rain. "Cities are just forests that forgot how to breathe," she concluded. "My job is to remind them."

The soft sounds of writing gave way to contemplative silence as each person completed their letter. Some folded their papers with origami precision, others let them remain open, ink drying in the evening air that carried temple bell echoes and the first moth wings of night.

Lachlan produced five boxes from beneath the table, each crafted from fallen cedar, their surfaces still bearing the texture of bark, the sweet scent of resin rising as he opened their lids. "These trees gave their bodies to hold your promises," he said, running a thumb along the grain that recorded decades of growth rings. "They know about patient time."

One by one, they placed their letters inside, along with the treasures gathered that morning—Sarah's stone nestled against pressed pine needles, Kenji's herbs wrapped in grandmother's teaching notes, Hana's willow twigs crossed like an artist's signature, Aisha's moss sample still damp with urban persistence. Each box received its contents like a reliquary, the wood seeming to warm under their touch.

The sealing wax appeared in a small brass pot,

heated over a candle flame until it ran red as maple leaves. Lachlan handed each person a seal carved with a different leaf pattern— ginkgo for Aisha, maple for Hana, oak for Kenji, pine for Sarah. As they pressed the wax, the leaf imprints emerged like fossils from the future, marking not just the boxes but the moment when intention crystallized into commitment.

"Open these in one year," Lachlan said, his own box already showing the patina of handling, evidence of his own forest promises kept and renewed. "When the forest seems distant. When concrete feels permanent. When spreadsheets multiply like invasive species. When galleries demand sterility. When prescriptions seem easier than plants. When permits get denied."

The final tea ceremony unfolded in movements refined by a thousand years of practice, but the hands that performed it bore new calluses— from pressing bark, from sketching with charcoal, from planting seeds in hostile soil. The tea tasted of rain and earth and the particular sweetness that comes from sharing transformation with others who understand the price of change.

Moonlight finally found them through the paper screens, painting silver calligraphy across the table where five boxes sat like seeds waiting for the right season to open. The garden's night sounds grew louder—crickets and water and wind through bamboo creating the soundtrack for this particular goodbye that was really just another form of beginning.

They rose together, boxes cradled like newborns or dreams or the future itself. At the threshold where shoes waited to carry them back to distant cities, they paused in a circle that needed no words. The forest lived in their hands now—in Sarah's soil-scented fingers, in Kenji's medicine pouch, in Hana's charcoal dust, in Aisha's pocket full of permits.

Lachlan stood in the doorway as they departed, his whiskey flask catching moonlight like captured lightning. Somewhere beyond the garden, a nightjar called its liquid note, and he smiled knowing they would hear it now in sparrow songs and subway rails, in coffee shop chatter and gallery openings, in all the places where forests hide, waiting to be remembered.

The Continuing Journey

Dawn arrived as a master printer pressing ink through leaves, each perforation in the canopy stamping copper light onto forest floor parchment. Lachlan McGregor's boots disturbed the volcanic loam's perfect registration, his satchel's leather worn supple from twelve months of academic warfare. He paused where seven cedars formed a living airlock, fingers brushing the whalebone clasp Hiroshi had carved from a beached pygmy right whale's jaw. The smell of freshly printed journals rose from the bag's depths - acid-free paper and cedar oil bindings mingling with older ghosts of peat smoke and Yuki's disapproval.

"Dr. McGregor?" The voice came softened by fifty-three weeks of breathing exercises, though Sarah's corporate crispness lingered in the dental consonants. She emerged through shafts of angled light, her navy blazer sleeves rolled to accommodate forearms dusted with pine resin tattoos. The Patek Philippe that once monitored merger deadlines now dangled from a willow switch above her left breast, its face frosted with morning condensation.

Lachlan's knuckle tapped the nearest cedar in greeting. "Your tree's been busy," he observed, pointing to where Sarah's pine had extruded sap armor around the abandoned smartphone they'd buried last monsoon season. The device's silhouette showed through translucent amber like a fly in Jurassic-era resin, cellular towers fossilized mid-transmission.

Kenji approached with the rolling gait of a man no longer rationing breaths, his grandfather's herb pouch swinging empty save for three persimmon leaves pressed during their final Kyoto session. The elm he'd befriended leaned conspiratorially over the trail, its lowest branch bearing the polished scar where he'd once hung IV bags of saline solution as humidity offerings. When he pressed his nose to the cambium layer, the tree released a puff of mugwort-scented pollen that turned his bow into involuntary laughter.

"You're early," Hana accused, though the charcoal smudges beneath her nails suggested she'd been sketching since moonrise.

Herwillow's branches dipped to catch the leather portfolio slipping from her shoulder, catkins brushing security tags from the Mori Art Museum's spring collection gala. The motion scattered charcoal dust across her Thom Browne trousers in patterns mirroring the tree's shadow script on nearby stones.

Aisha's arrival crackled with contained energy, her ginkgo sapling now wearing last winter's sidewalk concrete like a warrior's pauldron. She knelt without removing her Prada mules, fingers tracing the crack where steel rebar tendons merged seamlessly with xylem. "He's incorporated the subway vibrations," she marveled, cheek pressed to bark that pulsed faintly with the Yamanote Line's morning rhythm.

Lachlan waited until the forest stilled - seven nuthatches settling on seven branches - before unbuckling his satchel. The journal emerged wrapped in dyed mulberry paper, its binding threaded with cherry bark strips from their farewell ceremony. "The University of Chicago Press sends their... let's call it reluctant admiration," he announced, peeling back layers to reveal the embossed title: *Dendrochronology of Healing: Bridging Forest Wisdom & Immunological Markers*.

196

Sarah's index finger hovered over a diagram mapping pine phytoncides to reduced cortisol spikes, her corporate-nurtured need for quantification momentarily overriding forest etiquette. "You kept the Tokyo cohort data in?"

"Page forty-three," Lachlan confirmed, watching Kenji's reaction to an illustrated cross-section of his elm's bronchial-like vascular system. The younger man's throat worked soundlessly as his fingers traced labels detailing histamine-inhibiting terpenes.

A moth-eaten silence settled while pages turned in sync with maple leaves overhead. Hana froze at a full-page reproduction of her willow sketch from their third session, academic captions boxing her chaotic charcoal strokes. She touched the margin note - *Fig. 9: Artistic Output Correlating With Measured Cortisol Decreases* - and laughed with the bitter clarity of gallery rejections transformed.

"Does the text mention?" she began, but Lachlan was already unfolding the back flap to reveal her name in citations. The willow chose that moment to drop a catkin across the footnote about negative space's therapeutic merits.

Aisha's architectural assessment came sharp and pleased: "You've structured it like urban green corridors - clinical studies branching into case histories." Her finger bridged a gap between chapters. "Here's where readers switch from skeptical to invested."

The forest exhaled through twenty-three thousand stomata as they regrouped beneath Lachlan's cedar. His forehead pressed the bark's vertical seam where Hiroshi had once scored five marks for failed attempts at stillness. The old whiskey flask made its rounds, now filled with spring sap syrup that caramelized on the tongue like liquid dendrochronology.

Sarah's pine breathed its cinnamon benediction as she placed both palms against trunk flesh that outlasted stock markets. Kenji's elm deposited an antihistamine-rich leaf bundle in his upturned hat. Hana's charcoal found new purpose documenting the willow's assessment of her published work. And Aisha's ginkgo hummed a concrete-laced lullaby that shook loose municipal permit numbers from her hair.

They didn't notice the academic journal absorbing moss spores into its binding, nor the way shadows conspired to hide its ISBN barcode. The cedars remembered, as cedars do

- this communion required no peer review.

Sarah's hands moved with the dangerous grace of someone who'd retrained muscle memory - the same fingers that once orchestrated hostile takeover bids now arranging pine needle mandalas around a salvaged motherboard serving as incense holder. She lit three sticks of Kyoto sandalwood in the Dell logo's hollow, their smoke curling through gutted RAM slots that still whispered of midnight spreadsheet marathons.

"The CFO of Mitsubishi Heavy Industries hyperventilated during her first session," she confessed, positioning a dried chrysanthemum stalk to catch falling ash. "Turns out power ties restrict diaphragmatic movement." Her demonstration breath lifted the Botox-smooth space between her brows, pine resin sharpening air that once reeked of toner and ambition.

The group mirrored her intake - Kenji's lungs expanding beyond their former pharmaceutical limits, Hana's exhalation ruffling the MoMA catalog in her lap, Aisha's clavicle rising like a suspension bridge designed by enlightened engineers. Lachlan's pencil scurried across journal margins in glyphs borrowed from forest rangers and particle physicists alike.

"Now thank your adrenal glands," Sarah instructed, voice softening around the edges like overhandled stationery. "Then release their quarterly reports." Their collective exhale stirred the incense smoke into tornado patterns that briefly resurrected the ghost of her corner office before dispersing it through black pine boughs.

Kenji unfolded his tea ceremony like a medieval surgeon's kit - magnolia leaf wrappers, a mortar carved from lightning-struck oak, chamomile buds harvested from Chernobyl exclusion zone volunteers. His wrists rotated in the precise ellipses his grandfather used to grind sencha, though these motions now powered by regenerated cartilage rather than desperation.

"This one's half mugwort, half deleted emails," he joked, measuring leaves against a strip of bark paper scored with his childhood asthma metrics. The kettle - formerly his IV drip stand - sang a different pitch when filled with spring water, its vibration aligning with the elm's root system beneath their feet.

They drank from acorn caps lacquered with subway map patterns, the tea's bitterness cut by

200

wild honey from hives installed atop Sarah's former corporate headquarters. Aisha's hum of approval sent ripples across the surface tension, her tongue analyzing flavors like contract clauses. "You've balanced the urban particulates beautifully," she pronounced, tapping a nail against her cup's polymer coating.

Lachlan's notes spiraled into illegibility as steam transformed into temporary dendrites above the circle. "Remarkable," he murmured, though whether referring to Kenji's improved grip strength or the mycelial patterns in his own spilled tea remained deliciously unclear.

When the final sip drained, Sarah produced her old business cards repurposed as gratitude tags. "Write what you're ready to burn," she instructed, the thermal printer paper still bearing faint traces of emergency board meeting alerts. Kenji's characters flowed pharmaceutical-precise, Hana's stylus tore jagged glyphs, Aisha's fountain pen plotted infrastructure in iron gall ink. Their offerings smoked rather than burned - forest humidity preserving the words "mergers" and "metrics" just long enough for the pine to digest their meaning.

The ceremonial cough came from Lachlan's general direction, though his flask's position suggested alternative causes. "Your old assistant called last week," he mentioned offhand, watching Sarah track a ladybug's ascent up her former CEO desk bonsai. "Wanted your moonlighting policy for wellness retreats."

Her laugh unspooled a full octave lower than her investor pitch register. "Tell Amanda moonlight requires embracing shadows." The pine underscored her point by drizzling sap across the motherboard's last functional capacitor, fusing silicon and cellulose in permanent partnership.

Hana's sculptures emerged from the forest like mechanized saplings, copper arteries threading through willow withes in patterns that defied both Guggenheim curation and nature's usual schematics. She'd suspended the largest piece between three maples using tension cables stolen from bridge demolition sites, its rusted rebar fingers catching light that once spotlighted her failures in Chelsea galleries.

"This one breathes," she announced, tapping a hollow cedar branch that fogged intermittently

202

with the forest's humidity cycle. The group leaned close as lichen-encrusted gears ground out a melody matching the nearby stream's tempo, Hana's charcoal fingerprints visible on drive belts repurposed from Tokyo metro handstraps.

Aisha's blueprints unfurled with territorial majesty, vellum corners pinned down by bark strips still oozing medicinal sap. "Your willow's cousin in Shibuya," she indicated, tracing a green corridor that bypassed zoning laws using ginkgo growth patterns. The plans incorporated Hana's sculpture photos as elevation markers and Kenji's herb gardens as pollination waypoints.

Lachlan's laughter shook loose a mayfly from his beard. "You've weaponized municipal codes as if they're photosynthesis equations." His thumb smudged an elevation marker into something resembling Sarah's cortisol charts, the ink blurring into a nearby root system diagram.

They reconvened at the original cedar as dusk deployed its chromatic arsenal - indigo seeping through canopy gaps like spilled printer ink. Sarah's palms met bark first, her pine's circadian rhythm encoded in scar tissue that mapped twelve months of boardroom defections. Kenji's forehead pressed the northern face where Hiroshi's blade had once scored failure tallies, his breath fogging sap channels now publishing groundbreaking data.

When Aisha's blueprints rustled in the gathering wind, the cedar absorbed their arc through shadow puppetry on adjacent pines. Hana's sculptures clicked into harmonic convergence as their breathing synced to the forest's basal rate - six seconds in through Sarah's pine, eight seconds out through Kenji's elm, four second pause calibrated to Aisha's subway pulse.

"Not participants anymore," Lachlan murmured, his voice fraying at the dendrite level. The cedar translated his words into vascular tremors that bypassed eardrums for skeletal resonance. Somewhere beneath them, Tokyo's newest green corridor shivered into being along abandoned railway lines, its support beams already sporting the delicate lacework of Hana's signature oxidation patterns.

As fireflies switched shifts with bioluminescent fungi, the forest's approval registered in ways no journal could quantify - copper singing to cambium, cortisol metabolizing into chlorophyll, the relentless grid of cities finally learning to breathe in 7/4 time.

EPILOGUE

The forest remembers everything.

It remembers Lachlan McGregor's first stumbling steps off asphalt, the weight of failed peer reviews dissolving into cedar duff. It remembers Sarah's stiletto heels sinking into moss, her spreadsheet armor cracking like chrysalis. It remembers Kenji's inhaler abandoned beneath mugwort, Hana's gallery contracts becoming mulch, Aisha's permits transforming into prayer flags stretched between ginkgo branches.

Most of all, it remembers the moment when five humans stopped trying to measure mystery and began, finally, to breathe with it.

The journal sits on library shelves now, its pages slowly absorbing the particular humidity of academic archives. *Dendrochronology of Healing* - reviewers called it "groundbreaking," though they couldn't explain why reading it made them want to remove their shoes and press bare feet to earth. The data is solid, the methodology reproducible, the conclusions peer-reviewed into respectability.

But between the lines, in margins where science dissolves into poetry, the real story grows like moss on north-facing stones. It's in Sarah's boardroom, where executives now begin meetings with three minutes of breathing exercises. It's in Kenji's community garden, where former pharmaceutical patients learn to identify plantain by touch. It's in Hana's installations, where gallery visitors are invited to contribute twigs and stones to ever-evolving mandalas. It's in Aisha's vertical forests, climbing concrete walls one permit at a time.

And it's in the clearing where seven cedars still stand, their branches reaching across centuries to touch tomorrow. Where Hiroshi's bamboo chimes sing wind songs to anyone who remembers how to listen. Where a whiskey flask, long empty of alcohol, fills each dawn with dew that tastes of transformation.

The forest path remains, neither widening nor narrowing, neither easier nor harder to find. It simply waits, patient as growth rings, certain as sunrise, knowing that eventually, inevitably, other weary travelers will stumble from asphalt onto moss, their hands reaching for bark, their lungs remembering what it means to truly breathe.

The trees lean in, ready to whisper their secrets to anyone brave enough to press forehead to bark and count to 108. Ready to teach the only lesson that matters:

You were never separate. You were always home.

ACKNOWLEDGMENTS

To the cedars of Nikko, who taught me stillness. To the moss of Kyoto, who showed me softness. To the ginkgos of Tokyo, who demonstrated persistence. To Hiroshi, wherever you wander now, your bamboo chimes still sing. To all who trade spreadsheets for soil, galleries for groves, prescriptions for plants. To the forest in each of us, waiting to remember.

The author can be found most mornings pressed against a particularly patient oak, learning to count breaths in tree time. His whiskey flask now holds only rainwater and possibility.

THE END

ABOUT THE AUTHOR

Lachlan McGregor abandoned a promising career in cryptozoology to spend his days talking to trees and teaching stressed executives how to breathe. His previous academic work includes papers on Himalayan Yeti microbiota (retracted), dendrochronological anomalies in post-volcanic forests (ignored), and the therapeutic applications of forest bathing (finally, reluctantly, accepted).

He currently divides his time between Japan's ancient groves and whatever urban forest will tolerate his presence. His flask collection has been donated to various recycling programs, though he keeps one for "medicinal cedar infusions."

When not pressing his forehead against bark or teaching corporate warriors to identify moss species, he can be found annotating rejection letters with botanical diagrams or explaining to university administrators why his office hours are now held exclusively outdoors.He still can't explain the mechanism behind tree whispering. He's stopped trying.

AUTHOR'S NOTE

Written longhand in a forest clearing,
transcribed by candlelight

Dear Reader,

If you've made it this far, through twenty
chapters of humans pressing their foreheads
against trees and corporate executives learning
to breathe, then perhaps you understand
something that took me fifty-three years and
one spectacular career implosion to discover:
the forest has been waiting for us all along.

This story began, as many do, with failure. My
seventh grant proposal had just been rejected.
The phrase "lacks scientific rigor" had been
underlined twice in red ink—the academic
equivalent of a death sentence. I was sitting in
my climate-controlled office, surrounded by
data that proved nothing and journals that
measured everything except what mattered,
when I noticed the oak outside my window.

It had been there for two hundred years. It had
survived the construction of the university, the
paving of the parking lot, the installation of
security cameras that watched its branches for

"suspicious activity." And it was still growing, still breathing, still offering shade to students who never looked up from their phones.

I walked outside, dress shoes crunching across the manicured lawn, and did something I hadn't done since I was six years old: I hugged a tree.

Security found me there three hours later, tie loosened, shoes kicked off, forehead pressed against bark while I counted breaths in a language I didn't know I remembered. They asked if I needed medical attention. I told them I was conducting research.

In a way, I was.

What followed was two years of what my department chair called "academic suicide" and what I call learning to live. I traveled to Japan's forest therapy trails. I sat with salarymen who wept against cedars. I watched executives discover that spreadsheets couldn't calculate the value of silence. I learned that trees don't care about your impact factor, your h-index, or your tenure track.

They only care that you show up.

This novel is fiction, but every breath in it is real. Every tree has been touched. Every transformation has been witnessed. The data is accurate—cortisol does drop when we spend time among trees, natural killer cells do increase, communities with more urban forests do have lower rates of anxiety and depression. But the science, as Hiroshi would say, is just the gateway drug. The real medicine is something our instruments can't measure.

Some of you will read this and immediately need to find a tree. Good. Go now. Don't wait. Don't overthink it. Just go.

Some of you will read this and think it's all metaphorical, a pretty story about burnout and recovery dressed up in leaves. That's fine too. Metaphors are just truths wearing comfortable shoes.

And some of you—I hope many of you—will recognize yourself in Sarah's spreadsheets, Kenji's inhalers, Hana's rejected art, Aisha's buried homesickness. You'll see that the forest isn't asking you to give up your life, just to remember that you're alive.

The cedars I write about are still standing. The moss still grows on the north side of stones. The streams still sing in keys that bypass our ears and go straight to our bones. They're waiting for you, patient as always, ready to teach you the only curriculum that matters:

How to be human. How to be home. How to breathe.

If you find yourself in Kyoto, or Sydney, or Manhattan, or anywhere with a tree—and there's always a tree, even if it's struggling through sidewalk cracks—try this:

Press your palms against the bark. Count to 108. Listen.

What you hear might sound like wind, or traffic, or your own heartbeat. But if you listen closely, with your whole body, you might hear what the trees have been trying to tell us all along:

Welcome back. We missed you. You're right on time.

With muddy fingers and moss-stained knees,

Lachlan McGregor
Somewhere between the city and the forest
Always heading home

P.S. - My flask now holds collected rainwater from seven different forests. It tastes like memory and possibility. Hiroshi would approve.

READING GROUP GUIDE

Questions for Discussion

1.   Lachlan begins the novel as a failed academic clinging to scientific measurement. How does his relationship with empirical data evolve throughout the story? What remains of the scientist by the end?

2.   Each character has a different "breaking point" that brings them to the forest. Which resonated most with you? Have you experienced a similar moment of recognizing disconnection?

3.   The number 108 appears repeatedly—in breaths, in prayer beads, in bamboo notches. Research its significance in Buddhist and Hindu traditions. How does this number serve as a bridge between science and spirituality in the novel?

4.   Sarah's transformation from CEO to forest therapy guide might seem extreme. What makes her journey believable? What details show her changing relationship with control?

5.   Kenji carries his grandfather's wisdom while rejecting traditional medicine. How does the novel explore the tension between ancestral knowledge and modern healthcare?

6.   Hana's art evolves from rigid gallery pieces to collaborative forest installations. What does this suggest about creativity and

control? About the relationship between artist and environment?

7.   Aisha's story touches on displacement and the immigrant experience. How do her Ugandan roots inform her approach to Tokyo's urban forest? What does "home" mean in her journey?

8.   Dr. Blackwood represents institutional skepticism. Yet she too transforms. What finally convinces her? Is her conversion necessary for the story's message?

9.   The forest is almost a character itself. How does McGregor achieve this personification without falling into pure fantasy? What techniques make the trees feel alive?

10.   The novel critiques corporate culture, academic rigidity, and urban disconnection. Yet it avoids simple "nature good, city bad" dichotomies. How does it maintain this nuance?

11.   Discuss the role of failure in each character's growth. How does the forest reframe their professional "failures"?

12.   The whiskey flask evolves from coping mechanism to ritual object to rain collector. Trace its transformation. What does it symbolize?

13.   Many scenes involve physical touch—pressing against bark, bare feet on moss, hands in soil. Why is tactile experience so central to the characters' transformations?

14.   The ending suggests the characters will

return to their urban lives, changed. Is this realistic? Can transformation survive the return to routine?

15.   If you could spend 108 breaths with any tree from the novel, which would you choose and why?

Activities for Book Clubs

• **Forest Bathing Session**: Find a local park or forest. Spend 20 minutes in silence, phones off, simply being present with the trees.

• **Create a Nature Mandala**: Using found materials like Sarah does, create temporary art that will return to the earth.

• **Urban Nature Mapping**: Like Aisha, identify potential green spaces in your neighborhood. Where could nature reclaim concrete?

• **Breathing Practice**: Try the 108-breath meditation with a tree. Notice what arises without judgment.

• **Share Your Story**: When have you felt most connected to nature? Most disconnected? Share without trying to fix or solve.

ADDITIONAL RESOURCES

Books on Forest Bathing & Nature Connection

- *The Hidden Life of Trees* by Peter Wohlleben
- *Braiding Sweetgrass* by Robin Wall Kimmerer
- *The Nature Fix* by Florence Williams
- *Forest Bathing* by Dr. Qing Li

Scientific Studies Referenced

- Qing Li et al. (2007): "Forest bathing enhances human natural killer activity"
- Park et al. (2010): "The physiological effects of Shinrin-yoku"
- Morita et al. (2007): "Psychological effects of forest environments"

Organizations

- Association of Nature and Forest Therapy Guides
- International Society of Nature and Forest Medicine
- Children & Nature Network

Forests to Visit

- Nikko National Park, Japan
- Muir Woods, California
- Black Forest, Germany
- Białowieża Forest, Poland/Belarus
- Amazon Rainforest (while we still can)

A FINAL GIFT

Found tucked into the author's final manuscript

A Prescription from the Forest

Dosage: As needed, but daily recommended
No substitutions. No generics. No refills
necessary.

Instructions: Find tree. Any tree.
Remove shoes if possible.
Touch bark with both hands.
Breathe in for 4 counts.
Hold for 4 counts.
Breathe out for 6 counts.
Repeat until you remember.

Side Effects May Include:

- Sudden urge to cancel meetings
- Decreased tolerance for fluorescent lighting
- Spontaneous tree hugging
- Improved sleep patterns
- Mysterious sense of belonging
- Uncontrollable smiling at leaves
- Reduced need for coffee
- Increased awareness of seasons
- Strange desire to grow things
- Healing

Warning: Once you start listening to trees, you may find it difficult to stop. This is not a bug.

It's a feature.

Storage: Keep in heart at room temperature. Share freely. Effects increase when taken with others.

Expiration: Never. Trees have been offering this medicine for 370 million years. They're not stopping now.

End of manuscript

The forest continues

So do you

APPENDIX: Glossary of Terms

Japanese Terms

Shinrin-yoku (森林浴) - Literally "forest bathing." The practice of spending time in forests for therapeutic benefits. Developed in Japan in the 1980s as a response to tech-boom stress.

Ki no Sasayaki (木の囁き) - "Tree whispering." A meditative practice of pressing against trees to sense their energy, less scientifically documented than shinrin-yoku.

Kami (神) - Shinto spirits or phenomena worshipped in Japanese religion. Trees, especially ancient ones, are often considered to host kami.

Hinoki (檜) - Japanese cypress, considered sacred. Its oil has antimicrobial properties.

Sugi (杉) - Japanese cedar (*Cryptomeria japonica*). Despite the name, it's actually a cypress, not a true cedar.

Matcha (抹茶) - Powdered green tea used in Japanese tea ceremonies. Contains L-theanine, which promotes calm alertness.

Hōjicha (ほうじ茶) - Roasted green tea with a

distinctive brown color and nutty flavor.

Scientific Terms

Phytoncides - Antimicrobial volatile organic compounds emitted by plants and trees. From Greek "phyton" (plant) and "cide" (kill). Proven to boost human immune function.

NK cells (Natural Killer cells) - Type of white blood cell that plays a major role in rejecting tumors and virally infected cells.

Cortisol - Primary stress hormone. Elevated levels associated with anxiety, depression, and various health issues.

Terpenes - Large class of organic compounds produced by plants, especially conifers. Include pinene (pine scent) and limonene (citrus scent).

VOCs (Volatile Organic Compounds) - Organic chemicals that easily become vapors. In forests, these are often beneficial; in urban settings, often pollutants.

Cambium - Layer of cells between bark and wood where tree growth occurs.

Xylem - Tree tissue that transports water and nutrients from roots to leaves.

Phloem - Tree tissue that transports sugars

from leaves to rest of tree.

Mycorrhizal networks - Symbiotic associations between fungi and plant roots, allowing trees to share nutrients and even communicate.

Dendrochronology - Science of dating trees by their growth rings.

Botanical Terms

Cryptomeria japonica - Japanese cedar/sugi, endemic to Japan.

Ginkgo biloba - Maidenhair tree, one of the oldest living tree species.

Lenticels - Pores in bark that allow gas exchange.

Stomata - Pores in leaves for gas exchange and transpiration.

Sapwood - Younger, outer wood that transports water.

Heartwood - Older, inner wood that provides structural support.

Nurse log - Fallen tree that provides nutrients for new growth.

Epiphyte - Plant that grows on another plant

without parasitizing it.

Cultural/Spiritual Terms

Taniwha - Beings from Māori mythology that can take various forms, often guardians of specific places.

Mudra - Symbolic hand gesture used in Buddhism and Hinduism.

108 - Sacred number in Buddhism and Hinduism. Buddhist prayer beads have 108 beads. Represents completeness, the number of earthly temptations, or breaths in a meditation cycle.

Wabi-sabi (侘寂) - Japanese aesthetic finding beauty in imperfection and impermanence.

Medical/Psychological Terms

Piloerection - Hair standing on end, "goosebumps."

Erythema - Redness of skin from increased blood flow.

Vasoconstriction - Narrowing of blood vessels.

Bronchodilator - Medication that opens airways.

Antihistamine - Medication blocking histamine response in allergies.

GABA (Gamma-Aminobutyric Acid) - Neurotransmitter that reduces neuronal excitability, promoting calm.

Circadian rhythm - Natural internal process regulating sleep-wake cycle.

Ecological Terms

Biotic community - All living organisms in a particular area.

Allelopathy - Chemical inhibition of one plant by another.

Pioneer species - First species to colonize disrupted ecosystems.

Succession - Process of change in species structure over time.

Understory - Layer of vegetation beneath main canopy.

Duff - Partly decomposed organic matter on forest floor.

Loam - Fertile soil of clay, sand, and organic matter.

Academic/Research Terms

Impact factor - Measure of scientific journal's influence.

H-index - Measure of researcher's productivity and citation impact.

P-value - Statistical measure of evidence against null hypothesis. $P < 0.05$ typically considered significant.

Type II error - Failing to reject a false null hypothesis (false negative).

Peer review - Evaluation of work by others in same field.

Grant proposal - Application for research funding.

Tenure track - Academic career path potentially leading to permanent position.

Geographic/Cultural References

Kii Peninsula - Large peninsula in Japan, home to ancient pilgrimage routes and forests.

Nikkō - Mountain town north of Tokyo, famous for shrines and national park.

Yakushima - Island with ancient forest, inspiration for Princess Mononoke.

Tongariro - Volcanic area in New Zealand, sacred to Māori.

Waitākere Ranges - Forested hills near Auckland, New Zealand.

Urban/Architectural Terms

Green corridor - Connected green spaces allowing wildlife movement through urban areas.

Vertical garden - Garden growing on vertical surface, also "living wall."

Pocket park - Small park accessible to public, often in dense urban areas.

Brownfield - Previously developed land not currently in use.

Urban heat island - City area significantly warmer than surroundings due to human activities.

Measurement/Technical Terms

pH - Measure of acidity/alkalinity. 7 is neutral, below is acidic, above is alkaline.

Lux - Unit of illumination.

Hz (Hertz) - Unit of frequency, cycles per second.

BPM - Beats/breaths per minute.

RH (Relative Humidity) - Amount of water vapor in air as percentage of maximum possible.

Other Terms

Spectrometer - Instrument measuring properties of light.

Chromatography - Technique for separating mixtures.

Biomimicry - Design inspired by nature.

Phenology - Study of cyclic natural phenomena timing.

Ethnobotany - Study of relationships between people and plants.

Silviculture - Growing and cultivation of trees.

Note for Readers: Don't let unfamiliar terms stop your reading flow. Like the forest itself, this story reveals its meanings gradually, through context and experience rather than definition. Sometimes not knowing precisely is part of the journey toward understanding deeply.

Content:

228